Strategies in E...

STRATEGIES IN

Health Care Quality

Christopher R.M. Wilson, Ph.D.
Honorary Fellow, 1992–1994
University of Manchester

W.B. Saunders Company Canada Limited
Toronto Philadelphia London Montreal Sydney Tokyo

W.B. Saunders Company Canada
55 Horner Avenue
Toronto, Ontario
M8Z 4X6

W.B. Saunders Company
The Curtis Center
Independence Square West
Philadelphia, PA 19106

Strategies in Health Care Quality
ISBN 0-920513-12-3

Canadian Cataloguing in Publication Data

Wilson, Christopher R.M. (Christopher Richard Maclean), 1934-
    Strategies in health care quality

Includes bibliographical references and index.
ISBN 0-920513-12-3

1. Hospitals — Canada — Quality control.
2. Health facilities — Canada — Quality control.
3. Quality assurance — Standards — Canada.
I. Title.

RA971.W55 1992 362.1'1'068   C92-093733-0

Text/cover design/composition/technical art: Blair Kerrigan/Glyphics
Production: Francine Geraci

Printed and bound in Canada at Webcom

1 2 3 4 5   96 95 94 93 92

Dedication

A late graduation gift for
IAN LOUIS WILSON, B.A.
now in graduate school at
Old Dominion University,
who is fulfilling his promise.

Acknowledgements

There are many people whose assistance and friendship have supported the author in the development of this book. First and foremost is the Ontario Hospital Association. I retired on 30 April 1992 having completed fourteen years with the Association, which has been the cause of my learning about quality and governance, and the professional society that encouraged my writing. Few people have been so fortunate in the match between their talents and interests and the demands of their employer. Consulting for hospitals in Ontario under OHA's banner has been a privilege, full of meaning, friendships and enjoyment. Particular friends of this project at OHA have been Bill Barrable, Judy Moran-Fuke, John Tagg and Audrey Nelson.

In tackling the chapters on Medical QA I am indebted to a number of physicians: first to Hugh Carey, who pushed me to the point that I had to distinguish focussed studies from criterion audits; next to Donald Curtis, who believed that a non-physician had a contribution to make in assisting doctors to "do *their* thing." Kenneth Williams and Fulvio Limongelli have been valued teachers and friends, as has Spence Meighan, who has challenged and encouraged me throughout.

I acknowledge with pleasure the influence of three experts: Catherine Cornell in utilization review, David Brisley in risk management, and Beth Meuser, who is the author's unnamed teacher of CQI in Chapter 10.

Many of these people have read chapters and whole sections of this book, and have advised me on them, as have Margaret Hagerman, Joanne Watson and Janet Rouse, a management intern from the NHS, who came to work with me in Toronto on outcome indicators.

In March, I was appointed an honorary fellow of the University of Manchester, on the nomination of its Health Services Management Unit, for whom I teach QA in Britain.

My affiliation with the Schofields, the HSMU, and the University is the source of great pleasure.

I am much honoured by the Foreword contributed by Professor Evert Reerink, the dean of quality assurance in Europe, whose QA consortium in the Netherlands, CBO, has inspired a generation of QA leaders all over the world.

The book would not have been possible without Gerry Mungham, who wanted it for W.B. Saunders Company, Francine Geraci who, as editor, put it all together with affection, and Ronnie Bacher, who typed draft after draft, faultlessly. Important at various stages of the project was Carol Bonnett, my agent at MGA.

Thank you finally to my wife Louis, who directs a community agency, manages our home and financial affairs, and co-ordinates our sons' education. If authorship were a question of deserving, her name would be on the cover.

Christopher R.M. Wilson, Ph.D.
October 1992

Contents

Foreword

Sequelae are "in". This pertains to books, movies, and quality assurance alike. In our dynamic world things must move, and quality assurance is no exception.

Health care moves into new areas and needs fresh approaches to assessing and improving quality. Health care professionals require a change of language and fashion in order to stay interested and active in fields in which they have — by nature — little inclination. Enough reasons to welcome a comprehensive answer: the sequel to Dr. Christopher R.M. Wilson's *Hospital-wide Quality Assurance*. The change of times and the dynamics of the trade have been expressed in a completely updated and expanded book with a new title, the use of current and moderately aggressive language, the addition of new sections, an occasional blast towards attitudes worn out or belonging to the past, and an overall eminently readable text that will equally capture the minds of those who are already won for the cause and those who have their reservations.

Strategies in Health Care Quality will be read and used outside Canada as well. The Canadian health care system, a true hybrid with both American and European features, is the playground for this book. On both continents it will be ardently followed and wholeheartedly rejected. Such is the fate of any text on quality assurance in health care, and *Strategies* will be no exception. Canadians, Americans and Europeans will benefit from reading what the author, from his vast experience in the field, expresses in this text and conveys as his message: that which we call quality assurance "by any other name would smell as sweet".

Evert Reerink, MD, Ph.D.
Executive Director CBO, Utrecht
Professor of Quality Assurance in Health Care
Maastricht, The Netherlands

Part 1

Facility-Wide Quality Assurance

1

QA Yesterday, Today and Tomorrow

1.1
QA History

The publication of the 1983 *Standards for the Accreditation of Canadian Health Facilities* [1] was the watershed event for quality assurance (QA) in Canada. This manual did not invent QA, but it did name it and make it a universal expectation of hospitals. Even before 1983, many health facilities were implementing organized quality management: medicine and nursing departments had been conducting clinical audits and peer reviews since 1977, and prior to that, clinical laboratories, pharmacies, operating suites, radiology departments and other services had maintained strict quality control with the concurrent monitoring of standards. But 1983 put it all on the table. The *Standards* demanded that *all* organized departments have a QA program, that departmental programs share a generic likeness, and that their results be reported through the hierarchy to the hospital's governors, the board of trustees.

What has happened since the 1983 Surveyors' Conference, when the first QA *Standards* were unveiled, and today — nine years later, October 1992? And what can be said in response to that hardest of questions: How effective has QA been?

At a purely historical level, we can say that Canadian QA is now operating on its third definition of quality assurance. In 1983, QA was problem solving:

> *The essential components of the Quality Assurance program shall include: problem identification, problem assessment, implementation of measures to reduce or eliminate problems, and evaluation and monitoring of the effectiveness of implemented changes.*[2]

The ink on this paragraph was barely dry before the 1985 *Standards* were published, defining QA in terms of a comprehensive series of audits and reviews:

> *Quality Assurance is the establishment of hospital-wide goals, the assessment of the procedures in place to see if they achieve these goals and, if not, the proposal of solutions in order to attain these goals.*[3]

After some national health associations came out in favour of outcome indicators, the 1991 *Standards* flirted briefly with performance indicators before announcing accreditation's forthcoming marriage to continuous quality improvement (CQI).

While QA held centre stage, the Canadian Council on Health Facilities Accreditation (CCHFA) encouraged the articulation of other quality-related programs. Utilization review and management (URM) achieved major prominence in 1985, and risk management (RM) became a mandatory aspect of quality management in the 1991 *Standards*. In 1985, QA was extended to hospital boards of trustees, through the accreditation demand that boards subject themselves to external evaluation or engage in periodic, structured self-evaluation.

1.2
Effectiveness

Today, after Canada's nearly ten years of experience with the program, it is difficult to write about QA's effectiveness. The Council, its surveyors, administrators, physicians, QA co-ordinators, consultants like myself and, of course, line managers all know that QA has not, for all its promise, accomplished what we hoped it would. It has made some obvious gains, but it has also amassed some debts; we will look at both. My own involvement with QA has been so continuous that any criticism must carry a weight of self-incrimination. In the words of the ancient general confession, "We have done those things that we ought not to have done, and not done those things which we ought to have done." But fault finding seems inappropriate when we remember how many people have worked and studied and taught to make what looked so good become a reality. With this in mind, the correct starting point is QA's accomplishments. Four are clearly identifiable:

- *QA has raised the profile of quality of care.* In 1982, reporting quality was an unusual and specialized activity: only certain hospital departments and medical committees monitored what occurred and then advised authorities of their findings. Information prior to 1983 about quality of service or care tended to be negative and domestic. In those days, hospital managers knew far more about *dis*-quality than quality — about broken standards, negative incidents, patient complaints and complaints from other departments. Departmental quality information was domestic, i.e., unless the news was famous or notorious, reports of quality of care and service stayed within a given department. With the advent of QA, quality became news that had to be both shared and heard. This sounds so obvious today that, if any surprise is appropriate, it must arise over the secrecy about the hospital's and departments' main endeavours, which had so long been concealed.

This new awareness of quality has had several consequences. First, staff — for whom quality issues had commonly been a negative topic — had encouragement to promote, review, maintain and improve quality. Second, lay trustees — who had long been inhibited from talking about care issues — now had a source of information and structures through which they could question and understand what occurred. Third, management operating in a QA environment found opportunities to hear, and the means to do something about, quality problems. Fourth, the hospital's ability to account for quality occurred at a time when patients, payors and communities began to ask basic and insistent questions about the quality of care that *their* money was buying, that *their* hospital was providing.

- *QA has increased the ability of providers to question and measure quality of care and make both activities habitual.* Quality accountability has forced health care providers to develop skills and patterns of performance assessment. "Structure, process and outcome" has become a QA catchphrase. Everyone says it and most people know what it stands for: the alternative aspects of care or service activity that can be reviewed in QA. The term "audit", which prior to 1983 applied only to Nursing and Medicine, now applies to all provider departments — concurrently, if possible. Meanwhile, QA committees across the country have called on their departments to set up QA plans stating which indicators each will monitor and evaluate for the year. Department heads have become more sophisticated about data, sources, standards, surveys and norms.

- *Care and service have been improved because of the scrutiny of QA.* Prove it I can't, but I do believe it. After all, QA provides the essential ingredient to performance improvement: that is, the knowledge of present deficiencies. Even if all that is acknowledged is an enormous and long-term Hawthorne effect — i.e., that performance improves simply because it is under scrutiny — that still constitutes quality improvement. Nearly every department today can point to improved performance because of discoveries made in their pursuit of QA. These may not be technological breakthroughs or million-dollar cost savings, but they number in the thousands and have been important to the departments implementing them. QA has caused practitioners, supervisors and managers to sit on the same side of the table on quality issues, and that has become a powerful team.

- *QA has improved management practice.* Recently I challenged a group of CEOs and QA leaders to identify the benefits of ten years of QA in Canada. Their responses gave support to the benefits already described. In addition, they articulated three results that occurred in the management of a department's activity. They saw as beneficial the accreditation council's demand for the use of "principal functions", a term that encourages management to focus on a department's central and customer activities. But the increasing stress on outcome in the accreditation *Standards* and in the value system of QA have encouraged departments both to look at the effects of what they are accomplishing and to integrate service quality in management planning. Although documenting these effects would doubtless be difficult, their identification by a largely executive audience has added extra credibility.

But QA's critics must be given equal time. There are certainly three major issues: the high cost of diversity in implementation, opted-out physicians, and cost effectiveness.

High Cost of Diversity

Although critics would agree on the almost universal implementation of QA by hospitals, domiciliary facilities (e.g., nursing homes, homes for the aged), ambulatory care centres and public health programs, they also point to the immense cost of diversity in QA's implementation. There is no one Canadian model or handful of such models; with the exception of no more than ten per cent of programs that were implemented through outside consultants, nearly all other programs have been developed on site by staff who have read texts and attended conferences. This diversity is expensive for three reasons:

- The 1983 *Standards* created a new profession: QA co-ordinator, a full-time staff position in nearly every hospital of one hundred beds or more.

- QA is unevenly implemented given its home-made origins. No assumptions can be made about the quality of the QA program or of its practice.

- Without guidance and commonality, QA programs have tended to lay too heavy a burden on departments — i.e., if some reporting is good, more should be better. Where programs have demanded more measurement and reporting than can reasonably be provided by functioning departments, the quality of their reports has suffered, and their sense of alienation has increased.

Opted-out Physicians

If anecdotal reports are to be believed, the leading cause of the 2 + 1 accreditation awards (i.e., the resurvey of selected elements after one year, in order to achieve a three-year award) has been the lack of a medical QA program. Many QA co-ordinators and CEOs in Ontario will acknowledge that their hospital's medical staff QA program is moribund — except perhaps six months prior to a CCHFA survey. Chapters 5, 6 and 7 of this book will examine the issues surrounding medical QA. But two things must be said in criticism and in mitigation of QA. While physicians are still on the side of quality, the vast majority of them have no use for organized quality assurance. They find its demands inconsistent, time-consuming, bureaucratic and irrelevant to the improvement of care. On the other hand, we must remember that the first ten years of QA coincide with significant friction between physicians and governments, at least in Ontario. As hospitals became the protagonists' battleground, QA and other hospital duties for MDs suffered in the conflict.

Cost Effectiveness

The ultimate criticism of QA has been not that it is expensive, time-consuming, or a management demand (for all of these are true), but that it is ineffective: it does not accomplish legitimate and necessary goals. Its critics say that QA does not and cannot assure quality, and that for all its costs, structures, training and encouragement, hospitals do not and cannot point to better systems or improved care. Such critics cannot prove their negative assertions, but they can fault QA's supporters for not producing data that prove the value of all that they have promoted for a decade.

The Choice of CQI

Both the Joint Commission on the Accreditation of Healthcare Organizations (JCAHO) in the United States and the Canadian Council (CCHFA) have chosen a new beginning for the organization of health care quality. In 1988 the Joint Commission signalled its intent to promote continuous quality improvement (CQI) or total quality management (TQM). CCHFA followed suit with the introduction of continuous improvement language in its 1991 *Standards* and, more explicitly, in those for 1992.

It would not be unreasonable to suspect that both accrediting bodies had given up on QA themselves. The emergence of CQI/TQM in North American industry in the middle and late 1980s must have seemed like the answer to a prayer: here was a proven, effective, customer-oriented and

financially successful process to substitute for old QA, which
had been divisive, unpopular, costly and possibly ineffective.
The fact that they chose to begin anew (rather than augment
existing programs) speaks volumes for CCHFA's and
JCAHO's sense that QA was no longer salvageable. If this
interpretation is correct to any degree, their actions are a
heavy indictment of quality assurance.

The Survival of Quality Control

In spite of the negative assessment of quality assurance,
patients in both countries are still going to hospitals, being
cared for, getting better and going home. Employees are
going to work, working safely and living lives free from
injury. If quality assurance programs are not assuring and
promoting quality — and of course, hundreds of hospital
and thousands of departmental programs are doing just that
— then what is assuring quality of care?

There are two answers; one may be more of a surprise in
Canada than in the United States, where for years there has
been a strong regulatory interest in quality of care. The
bodies that promoted and inspected quality before QA are
still its effective allies nine years later. Although hospitals love
to criticize CCHFA, they don't criticize it very fiercely: they
know that its triennial surveys are the occasions when, right
across the hospital, deficiencies not addressed earlier are at
last put right or brought up to date. Professional societies,
from the physicians' Royal Colleges to member associations,
wield a major influence on individual practice at the highest
standard, as do health science faculties in universities and
colleges across Canada. The list of such agencies would have
to include free-standing bodies such as the Hospital Medical
Records Institute and the Canadian Standards Association, as
well as recognize the important contribution of the
provincial and local government programs and agencies that
inspect the environment and essential services, kitchens,
laboratories and imaging departments, labour practices and
resident accounts.

The second quality-support mechanism has been the hospitals' many quality control (QC) activities, most of which predated QA. QC has been well known in line departments: laboratory QC, radiation protection systems in imaging departments, narcotics control, daily balancing in Accounting, preventive maintenance in Plant Services, and scores more. As well, medical QC has been the purview of Medical Advisory committee (MAC) subcommittees — Tissue & Audit, Medical Records, Credentials, Pharmacy & Therapeutics, Infection Control and others. In the early days of QA, some saw QC as yesterday's leader. Instead, QC may prove to be the "man for all seasons".

1.3
Strategies in Health Care Quality

When the publishers asked me to update *Hospital-wide Quality Assurance* (*HQA*),[4] I suggested an entirely new text. With certain obvious exceptions, such as quotations from outdated accreditation *Standards, HQA* has not aged badly; it continues to be read and used in Canada and especially now in the U.K. Its main drawback is that it does not go far enough. New quality concepts have been developed in addition to the basic QA model promoted by the 1985 accreditation *Standards*. Because these elements were additions rather than substitutions, it was decided to leave *HQA* as the basic text that provides a conceptual framework for quality assurance and covers the political aspects of how to start, structure, direct and maintain the hospital-wide program. Building on this frame, the present book, *Strategies in Health Care Quality,*

- updates the definition of QA to 1992 (Chapter 2);

- introduces outcome indicators as an essential and practical QA tool (Chapter 3); and

- promotes four methods of assessing performance rather than just one — i.e., repetitive audits.

Part 2 is devoted entirely to medical quality assurance:

- Chapter 5 defines medical quality assurance with the benefit of an historical perspective;

- Chapter 6 deals with medical care appraisal; and

- Chapter 7 describes the discipline and tools of utilization review and management.

Part 3 consists of two chapters on risk management:

- Chapter 8 presents RM from the perspective of a line department;

- Chapter 9 describes the facility-wide program.

Part 4 contains three chapters that present continuous quality improvement (CQI):

- Chapter 10 describes CQI through its historical evolution and proposes how it would be structured in a facility;

- Chapter 11 deals with the development of a quality improvement project and presents the Seven Tools of CQI;

- Chapter 12 reviews the applicability of CQI to health care and proposes a sequence of steps to take a hospital from today's QA to tomorrow's CQI. Unsatisfied with the industrial model of CQI, I have presented a complementary model that accommodates both technical/professional quality and customer service quality.

1.4
The Management
of Quality

I would like to conclude this introductory chapter with two recommendations that apply regardless of whether the topic is QA 1992, utilization review, risk management, or CQI/TQM. The first is the necessity for all these programs to be led from the top. The second is to keep them simple and unencumbered.

Find the Captain

Why are there very few CEOs among the membership of the Canadian Association of Quality in Health Care? Why is QA leadership vested in a junior manager and not a vice president or assistant executive director? We are accustomed to the realization that medical staffs have not bought into QA, but has no one noticed that CEOs have not either? They want and need it to work; they would like it to be more useful and less boring, but few CEOs have adopted their facility's QA program or given it their direct vital attention. Of course, this is not true of all CEOs. Several excellent ones spring to mind whose commitment has made the hospital's program their program.

Last November the *1992 Schedule of Professional Development Opportunities*,[5] sponsored by the Canadian College of Health Service Executives, was delivered to my office. The College's program would have been chosen carefully to reflect its view of what is likely to be interesting and important to its members, because programs are intended at least to pay for themselves, and if possible, to show a profit. Among these twelve program titles (Exhibit 1.1), there is no mention of 1991's hottest topic:

CQI. Nor do the program descriptions mention quality in any form. The conclusion is not that the College is out of touch; quite the contrary. The fact is that, when it comes to quality, Canadian CEOs are on the sidelines.

Exhibit 1.1
1992 Schedule of Professional Development Opportunities

---

1. Feb. 6-8   "Decision Making That Values Differences"
                  National Health Care Ethics Forum

2. Feb. 20-21   Professional Advancement and Review Workshop

3. Feb. 23-25   "Downsized — Not Capsized"
                  Winter Management Conference

4. April 5-7   Spring Management Conference
                  (Downsizing, Mergers and Bill 120 in Quebec)

5. May 3-5   CEO Leadership Institute

6. June 7-9   CCHSE Annual National Conference
                  (Focus: Creativity, Innovation and Lateral
                  Thinking)

7. June 10   Third Annual Conference on Ambulatory Care

8. Sept. 24-26 Utilization Management Congress

9. Oct. 27-28   Professional Advancement and Review Workshop

10. Oct. 28-30   Fall Management Conference

11. Nov. 15-17   "Nursing Administration: Positioning for Power"
                  Nursing Management Conference

12. Nov. 20-22   "Getting It All Together"
                  (CEO/Board Retreat)

13. Dec. 3   Corporate Members' Program

    — Sponsored by the Canadian College of Health Service Executives.

The issue here is not a matter of delegation but a lack of involvement in — or an ambivalence towards — quality of care. It is inconceivable for a CEO to be *not* intimately involved with the hospital's financial system, *not* constantly in touch with the chief financial officer, and *not* demanding of subordinates that they respond appropriately to periodic reports and variances. Do quality reports receive the same attention and excite similar leadership behaviour? Yes, in some places; but in total, very rarely.

As so often, the present situation is explicable chiefly in terms of the past. QA began with the professionals who had in fact been doing it all along: nurses, pharmacists, laboratory technologists and others. It made sense for facility-wide programs to come together around those who knew what they were doing. Still today, QA in Canada belongs to department staff and their manager, to a QA committee composed largely of middle managers, and to a QA co-ordinator who is their peer. While QA data should be reported in line to the department's vice president or equivalent, the latter is often uncomfortable about receiving the data, and uncertain what to do with them when they are presented.

Senior management's avoidance of clinical responsibility has been costly to the facility's QA program. Carroll was writing about QA in the United States in 1984, but her words sound as though they were written for Canadian QA in 1992:

> *A list of the faults commonly found in hospital quality assurance would include the following observations:*
> 1. *There is no identifiable central body that is responsible for and authorized to direct hospital-wide quality assurance activities.*
> 2. *Quality monitoring and control responsibilities and duties are fragmented throughout the organization.*
> 3. *There is little or no communication with respect to review plans, study findings, or corrective measures among the many organizational units. This is particularly apparent in the case of the medical staff, which typically fails to share quality monitoring findings with other organizational units.*

4. *There is no clear assignment of authority for the implementation of corrective actions at any level of the structure or within the various organizational units.*[6]

Paying for Excess Baggage

The Evaluation Inventory and the QA Schedule listed in Exhibit 1.2 come from two medium-sized acute hospitals (200–400 beds) in Ontario. All the items listed in the Exhibit were listed on the documents named; however, I have rearranged them to show concurrence between the lists and grouped them according to the probable purpose of each entry. Two features should strike the reader: first, the sheer size of the list; and second, the heavy load of management and human resources provisions that have become stated components of these QA programs. Although these are only two of such lists in my possession, I believe them to be fairly typical of developed programs, and particularly those that have been enhanced by management.

Exhibit 1.2
Components of Departmental QA programs Expected by Two Hospitals in Ontario

Hospital A The Evaluation Inventory	Hospital B The QA Schedule
Management Practice	
Departmental goals — Annual objectives	
Policies and procedures	Policies and procedures
Terms of reference for dept. committees	
Dept. meetings documented	Dept. meetings documented
	Monthly statistics
	Staff utilization review
	Operating budget
	Capital equipment budget

Human Resources Activities

Job descriptions
Orientation program
Performance appraisals   Performance appraisals
Continuing education available
                                          Annual certification
                                          Delegated medical acts

Risk Management Provisions

Equipment maintenance program   Equipment maintenance program
Annual fire education
Annual disaster plan review
                                          Incident reports
Infection control procedures   Infection control procedures

QA Program

Mission statement
Principal functions
Daily monitors
QA reporting — Feedback to staff
QA planning
Standards development
QA binder

Quality Assessment

Pt./client feedback
Chart audits   Chart audits
Documentation of pt. teaching   Documentation of pt. teaching
                                         Therapy audits:
                                                 4 procedures: per mo. — 10
                                                 3 incidents: all occurrences
                                                 6 procedures: per mo. — 6

This inappropriate growth has three severe consequences. First among these is the loss of focus. In all of the items in the two schedules illustrated, where is the real QA — or is it all QA? After all, most of these items occur in the accreditation manual, somewhere. The second consequence is the quality of response. The inevitable consequence of increasing the volume and variety of demands in QA is to impair the quality of the evaluation of performance and the reports based on it. Third is the loss of ownership. QA activities have become primarily a management function, a more detailed and time-consuming system of accountability. They have lost their relationship to staff performance or patient satisfaction or outcome. The importance of the questions addressed in QA has deteriorated. QA has alienated its natural allies. Health care practitioners who have always had strong motivation and pride in performance have seen QA come to them and then be snatched away by management.

In order to help QA leaders cope with the problem of what belongs in the QA program and what does not, I have proposed what I call (after Jaques[7]) the Requisite Rule. This states that, in order to be included in the essential quality assurance program, each structure, practice, and written formulation must be judged requisite or necessary to:

- *either* the department head in his or her management of the quality of the department's performance

- *or* senior management in the discharge of its duty to be accountable for quality to the hospital's board of trustees.

The effective quality assurance program is a partnership between line departments, which manage quality, and senior management, which accounts for it to the board. The partners have complementary roles: the one monitors, measures, maintains and manages quality of care and service concurrently and prospectively; the other determines what quality the facility should achieve, provides funds or resources to that level, and accounts for this to the board.

The QA program's two foci are management of performance and accountability for results. Therefore, whatever structure or obligation is not essential to one or both of these goals should *not* be considered part of the QA program.

There are three caveats. First, the department heads determine what they need for the management of quality. Senior management should not saddle them, for the sake of uniformity, with quality management systems legitimately required by other departments. QA programs in Radiology and Social Services should be different in emphasis and content, while still using the same generic forms. Second, senior management should understand that the Requisite Rule is intended to limit management's power to increase the demands of the QA program — the limit being what management actually requires in order to account for quality. Third, the model has nothing to say about the appropriateness of all sorts of other management practices and the necessity for other information systems. However, it recommends that they all be justified on their own merits, and not as a part of the QA program. In past attempts at comprehensiveness, QA programs have lost their essential bifocal nature.

If senior management were to adopt the Requisite Rule for its facility, it might achieve a program that demonstrates certain attributes. That is to say, QA programs should be:

- *Lean*. QA can be low in cost and require little extra time, low structure, minimum paper. The ideal is efficient monitoring with consistent improvement.

- *Specific*. QA should be a tightly focussed program. It should exist alongside, but be separate from, the MIS and Human Resources systems, and the management practice requirements of the facility.

- *Action-oriented*. The program needs to focus on outcomes, to be inventive rather than routine, and to value inquiry over recording.

- *Department-driven.* QA should be based on what the department or program needs to do to maintain and improve quality.

- *Negotiable.* Executives who must account for quality should negotiate their demands with those who do QA.

- *Built on trust.* The hospital is a team. Senior managment serves line departments. Effective programs help rather than censure.

- *Client-focussed.* All departments have a client, either an internal client (another department) or an external client (usually, the patient). Quality assurance should begin and end with the client. If it doesn't matter to the client, how much can it matter to staff?

References

1. Canadian Council on Hospital Accreditation (1983). *Standards for the Accreditation of Canadian Health Facilities.* Ottawa: CCHA.
    The title *Standards* is used throughout this text to denote the manuals developed from time to time by the Canadian Council on Health Facilities Accreditation (CCHFA) or its predecessor, the Canadian Council on Hospital Accreditation (CCHA). These manuals have been called, at different times, *Guide to Accreditation* (1972, for example) and *Standards for the Accreditation of Canadian Health Care Facilities* (1986). Today they come without a lead title: one 1992 manual is called simply, *Acute Care — Small Community — Hospitals 1992.*
2. *Ibid.,* p. 43.
3. Canadian Council on Hospital Accreditation (1985). *Standards for the Accreditation of Canadian Health Facilities.* Ottawa: CCHA, p. 45.
4. Wilson, C.R.M. (1987). *Hospital-wide Quality Assurance.* Toronto: W.B. Saunders.
5. Canadian College of Health Service Executives (1991). *1992 Schedule of Professional Development Opportunities.* Ottawa: CCHSE.

6. Carroll, J.G. (1984). *Restructuring Hospital Quality Assurance: The New Guide for Health Care Providers.* Homewood, IL: Dow-Jones Irwin, pp. 31-32.
7. Jaques, E. (1989). *Requisite Organization: The CEOs' Guide to Creative Structure and Leadership.* Arlington, VA: Cason Hall.

2

Quality Assurance and the PIER Model

Differing Reflections in the Water

Few activities have presented so many successive different faces as what is now called quality assurance (QA). The basis for each of these faces has been the need for those providing patient care to examine and account for the care they are giving. In 1983 QA was seen as problem solving; in 1985 it was the continuous validation of performance against goals. In Canada, the Canadian Council on Health Facilities Accreditation (CCHFA) defines QA, and in their 1992 *Standards* a new face emerges. The new definition is, "performance monitoring leading to real improvement". Health care organizations must now meet the current accreditation standards, and expand their programs from the trail of audits practised from 1985 to 1990 into the more dynamic program sought in 1991 and 1992. This chapter, based on the text of the 1992 *Standards*, tells how this can be done.

The 1992 *Standards* are a useful base from which to begin because they are at once generic, in that they use the same text for all departments, and general, providing a

model applicable to any health system, community health
facility or hospital, in Manitoba or Britain. In addition, the
1992 *Standards* announce the arrival of continuous quality
improvement (CQI) in Canadian health facility management.
CQI — or its synonym, total quality management (TQM) —
is expected to enjoy a long run.

2.1
The Organization
of Quality
Assurance

The 1992 QA Standard

The quality assurance standard statement reads:

> . . . *[The Department] has planned and systematic*
> *activities for monitoring and evaluating the quality of*
> *patient care/service, including a plan for action(s) and*
> *follow-up to ensure that the action(s) is effective in*
> *continually improving the quality of care/service.*
> *(CCHFA, 1992)*

Quality assurance has three purposes, two of which are
named in this standard statement. The first is the
department's historic responsibility *to manage* the quality of
the product or service that is provided by the department or
team ("monitoring and evaluating. . . and follow-up").
Second is the obligation *to improve* quality by eradicating
poor performance and seizing opportunities to improve.
The third purpose of QA, which will be reviewed with
reference to Clause 9 below, is the obligation *to account* for
the quality of the department's care and service.

> *Clause #1. There are quality assurance activities in place which support the facility-wide quality assurance program.*[1]

In order to achieve these three purposes the QA program needs to be "planned and systematic". Canada's first QA *Standard* defined QA as problem solving (CCHA, 1983). The 1985 *Standard* stressed the need for QA to be continuous and comprehensive. The 1992 *Standard* maintains this focus. A department's QA program needs to be planned, and the plan must match the QA plan of the facility (Clause 1). It must also be systematic, as prescribed in Clauses 4 through 7.

Direction and Participation

> *Clause #2. There are clearly assigned responsibilities for quality assurance within the service.*

> *Clause #3. There is broad involvement of staff in quality assurance activities.*

Clauses 2 and 3 complement each other. They say, in effect, that the QA program must be managed effectively, with designated individuals taking responsibility for its different activities. At the same time, broad staff participation is expected. I have translated Clause 3 to mean that all staff at all levels, within a department, should participate in a QA activity every year. I am sure this is the goal departments should aim for. It should be remembered that of all the activities that make up the QA program — choice of audit topic, development of standards, checklists and questionnaires, gathering data, analyzing results, and planning remedial action — only reporting is specifically a management function. The possibilities for staff participation are legion, but it does mean that the QA enterprise be anticipated and planned, and not cobbled together at the last moment.

Keeping Score

> *Clause #8. There is documentation to support all quality assurance activities.*

In the army the new recruit is told: "If it moves, salute it; if it doesn't, whitewash it." I am reminded of this maxim, which I first heard forty years ago, in acknowledging quality assurance's obsession with paper. Everything is committed to paper; nothing is discarded. We have standards and criteria, minutes of meetings, quality control checklists, studies, print-outs, and data, data, data. Then, quite sensibly, people begin to worry about confidentiality and, in some jurisdictions, the discoverability of all this data by subpoena. If no one else, the QA committee must address this problem and develop sensible guidelines for both confidentiality (i.e., the anonymity of patient, care giver and evaluator) and the creation and retention of data by departments.

People ask, How long should we keep QA data? Because it is not primary data (charts, reports, consults, etc.), there is no obligation to keep it at all. However, for practical reasons, staff should keep QA data until the next accreditation survey, and audit data until the audit is repeated, for purposes of comparison.

Providing Feedback

> *Clause #9. The results of the quality assurance activities are communicated within the service, to management and to relevant staff and services according to the reporting timetable. Staff receive feedback from management on the information transmitted.*

This clause offers four points of advice:

- The first people who have an interest in the department's results, and the right to know them, are the staff. Feedback should be immediate, given to all shifts, graphic if possible, and posted, where confidentiality allows.

- Second, accountability for quality is owed to management. While the CEO or vice president need not become a QA expert, he or she must receive and render account for the quality of care, products and services achieved by each reporting department. This responsibility cannot be sloughed off to a QA committee.

- Third, while QA has been very good at passing messages up the line, few programs have developed mechanisms for providing feedback to departments. When it is remembered that most departments will not be required to report their QA results more frequently than quarterly, it is not unreasonable to expect senior management to respond formally (with recommendations and follow-up questions) at least twice a year.

- Fourth, departments have an obligation to share their results with co-operating or interfacing departments. Quality improvement reminds us that every worker and, by the same token, every department is a client of another and a service provider to a third party. Each department needs to evaluate what it receives from another, whether it be products, people or data, and should provide feedback on its satisfaction or dissatisfaction with what it receives. Similarly, the department has an obligation to share its data, warts and all, on the quality of its product or service with the department or other client whom it serves.

2.2
Program
Management
and QA
Committees

The *Standards* are silent about the existence of or need for a
QA committee. This is a reminder that the QA committee is
a local structure rather than a universal requirement.
Personally, I cannot conceive that a facility or agency could
operate an effective program without involving such a group
or groups. QA committees, all of whom share the same
functions, occur at various levels of the organization. Large
departments often constitute a committee to ensure
participation of all levels of staff and sections of the
department in its QA activities. Frequently, CEOs of small
hospitals will create a QA committee to manage the facility-
wide program for them. Sometimes, and very sensibly, senior
management itself will constitute the QA committee and
devote specific time at its regular meeting to the accounting
for and management of quality and the QA program. Some
facilities that adopt this practice will convene a subsidiary
committee to maintain commonality between the QA
practised in the facility's several divisions.

Medical staffs have frequently constituted special QA
committees that report to the Medical Advisory committee.
Ontario's *Prototype Hospital By-laws* recommended this
practice.[2] Medical leaders have not been prepared to see the
Tissue & Audit committee undertake responsibility for QA
in addition to its historic and well-defined quality control
role.

Finally, there is, or should be, a QA committee of the
board. Although some Joint Conference committees have
been pressed into this role, experience suggests that this has

not been the best answer. The QA committee of the board needs to have a clear majority of lay trustees. While as much as seventy-five per cent of its agenda should be patient related, including risk management and utilization review, significant attention also needs to be given to the facility's support services and data departments. Neither of these stipulations is natural to a Joint Conference committee.

I have discussed the membership and activities of these committees elsewhere.[3] Neither time nor experience has changed my mind as to the helpful — or rather, essential — roles they can play within the facility-wide program.

2.3
Providing
Assurance of
Quality

The PIER Model

The foregoing paragraphs provide the organizational context for the QA program. It is time now to describe the nature and method of quality assurance itself.

Quality assurance is an information system that allows a department to answer on a repeat basis two questions: How well is the department doing its job? and, How do we know?

The information system is focussed exclusively on the interface between the service provider — the department — and its client, who may be the patient or another customer. Thus, QA should be interested primarily in outcome and output rather than their antecedents (structure and process) and on the work of the service providers, whether general staff or practitioners, rather than management.

The starting point for QA, then, is the definition of the

job whose performance the system will measure. A useful term introduced in *Hospital-wide Quality Assurance* and now in the CCHFA *Standards* is the *principal functions* (Standard Area I.2) of the department. Principal functions are to QA what a job description is to performance appraisal: the basis for discussing performance. Principal functions name the major activities or divisions in the department's work. As such, usually they are too extensive to evaluate in their entirety, and QA must subdivide them into *important components.*

The heart of quality assurance is the *measurement of performance.* Various methods are used to assess the department's performance (of important components of its principal functions); four will be described. But evaluation can never be the end of the story in QA, which is an action strategy; departments must complete the loop by acting upon or responding to what they discover about their performance. The current imperative in QA is to remedy, certainly, but always strive to improve the department's performance.

The accreditation *Standards* describe four steps or constructs that constitute a simple and practical sequence or model of quality assurance:

- the *planning* of QA with reference to *principal functions;*

- the *identification* of *performance indicators/important components,*

- the *evaluation* of performance; and

- *response* to findings by *remedying, revising and reporting.*

This sequence is known as the PIER model: planning, identification, evaluation and response. The acronym also stands for principal functions, indicators/important components, evaluation, and the "three Rs": remedy, revise, report.

Principal Functions

In beginning the PIER model with principal functions, we are reaching all the way back to the first of the accreditation *Standards*: the demand that all departments have a mission, principal functions, goals and objectives. Standard 1, Clause 2 reads: "There is a written description of the principal functions of the service." It is most appropriate that QA should be anchored to the *raison d'être* of the service and that assurance be provided on the quality of the department's performance of its authorized mission or role. Thus, when I am asked to assist in the introduction of QA or implementation of the PIER model, my first instruction to the gathering of department heads is:

"Write a one- or two-sentence (mission) statement beginning: The role of my department is. . . ."

Following this, the instruction will be:

"Now I want you to identify your department's principal functions."

Having lived principal functions for four years, as they have been the foundation of all my teaching and model building in QA, I am still often surprised by the construct. After a long day teaching in London, in which I had reviewed a number of QA ideas and strategies with British managers, I asked them to select just one idea that they thought would be of special value in their program back home. More than sixty per cent of them had written independently, "principal functions". People like to use them because, to quote Dr. Samuel Johnson, they concentrate the mind wonderfully. Principal functions provide departments with a basic structure on which they can organize their QA. They show clearly what needs to be assessed and what does not. They are the department's first handle on managing quality.

The second surprise is that the task of identifying and establishing principal functions is more sophisticated and difficult than I generally remember. Yet there should be no surprise; after all, the demand is to summarize the essential work of the department in twenty words or less! The department's role statement answers the question: What contribution to its function and mission does the facility expect from your department? Principal functions are the answer to the next question: What activities does your department engage in, in the fulfillment of its role? Of course, departments do all sorts of things, and herein lies the difficulty. How do you sort the important from the unimportant? What does "principal" mean; i.e., how important does the activity need to be to make the list?

Some of the rules we have adopted provide a structure to the task and make it somewhat easier. The following are the most useful guidelines:

- A principal function is an *activity* and not a goal. It is something that staff actually do. I sometimes use the line: If I caught your people doing their jobs, what would I find them doing?

- A principal function leads to an *outcome,* that is, a product or service. It has a client outside of the department.

- For these reasons, there are two disqualifications. A principal function is *not* done by management but by staff. This leads to the second: A principal function is *not* a maintenance activity, i.e., any one of a host of highly necessary management activities that support the work of the department, such as budgeting, staffing, or staff education.

- Principal functions should be expressed in lay language, naming the function, using an active verb.

- A satisfactory list will consist of four to six functions and will encompass eighty to ninety per cent of the department's workload. Listing fewer than four functions does not differentiate the department's activities in enough detail to provide a basis for planning. Departments offering more than six functions are encouraged to group similar activities so that they have a manageable list.

Readers are invited to review the lists of principal functions given in Chapter 3, with reference to indicators (Exhibits 3.11 to 3.16). Principal functions were discussed in some detail in my earlier book.[4] However, there is one issue that comes up frequently and is not addressed elsewhere: the relevance of the nursing process to principal functions.

When asked to list principal functions, nurse managers on both sides of the Atlantic often resort to the four elements of the nursing process: assessment, planning, implementation and evaluation. But it does not make sense to separate assessment from planning; implementation is not a specific enough term — it is the whole meal in one bite; and evaluation is not a formal function but a reassessment of the patient and clinical situation following intervention. To use the nursing process as the principal functions is also to misunderstand the essential purpose of the concept, which was to prevent the division of the nursing role into a list of disconnected skills or activities: bed baths, dressings, charting, teaching, medications, etc. All these activities will, from time to time, be part of the nurse's role, but all are carried out in the context of the nursing process. In this sense the nursing process is not another activity or set of activities, but a strategy to integrate all patient care activities. The nursing process is in fact the *universal standard* for all activities. Individual nursing tasks can be targetted for performance review as long as all assessments begin with the question: Was (or, How was) the nursing process utilized in the provision of care?

Important Components

> Clause #4. *The important components of the service are identified and provide the focus for quality assurance activities.*
>
> 4.1 *The important components are derived from the principal functions of the service.*

> 4.2   *Priority is given to components of the service that are:*
> - *outcome-related*
> - *interservice*
> - *high-risk*
> - *high-volume*
> - *problem-prone.*

The term "important component" was introduced to the QA lexicon in the 1991 *Standards.* In arriving at performance indicators, departments were instructed to:

- identify the important components of their principal functions;

- set performance standards for each important component; and

- select indicators to measure their degree of achievement.[5]

What soon became apparent was that "important components" was a construct or concept whose usefulness was not limited to indicator development. Important components are the working unit of QA. Most principal functions are too large in volume and scope to be appropriate subjects of an audit or other assessment. Important components focus down to an activity that can be reviewed with clear definition.

In identifying important components, managers must remember that they are just principal functions writ small. Important components are still activities identified by name; as the term implies, they are identifiable components of the principal activity or function. Some examples will help. The Food Service manager may identify the preparation of soups, entrées, desserts, beverages, salads and sandwiches as important components of the principal function, "food preparation". Other examples are given by department in Exhibit 2.1.

Exhibit 2.1
Important Components of Some Common Principal Functions

Department	Principal Function	Important Components
Nursing (Surgical Unit)	Treatment	Administration of medications IV therapy Wound care Pain control
Medical Records	Transcription	Consultations Discharge summaries Radiology reports
Engineering	Maintenance	Preventative maintenance program Maintenance calls Shop repairs/Equipment
Social Work	Crisis Intervention	Patient support Assessment Liaison with care givers Professional referral

Performance Indicators

Important components notwithstanding, the "I" in the PIER model stands for indicators. Explicit performance indicators are difficult to identify; thus, it is not inappropriate to target them in a model. More important, good indicators are sensitive to changes in performance and are highly efficient to use in monitoring and assessment. Further, indicators are a construct used in risk management and utilization review, and are central to monitoring in CQI.

As indicator development and use is the sole topic of Chapter 3, I will not attempt to discuss it here. For now, I offer a simple definition: An indicator is a quantity that tells you something about quality. It is always a number — either a raw score or a rate of occurrence. It is related to the performance of the hospital as a whole ("global indicators"), to the experience of the patient, or to aspects of professional performance.

Indicators occur twice in the PIER model: once in relation to their identification and, in the U.S., their testing or validation. Second, indicators are treated as one of four major sources of data used in QA evaluation.

Evaluation

> *Clause #5.   A process is established for evaluating the important components of the service.*
>
> 5.1   *The process includes:*
> *   *establishment of the desired or expected level(s) of performance for each important component of the service.*
> *   *selection of criteria or indicators to measure the degree of achievement against the expected level(s) of performance.*
> *   *determination of the actual level of performance through collection of data.*
> *   *analysis of data.*

For several reasons, Clause 5 is a confusing prescription to follow. The opening sentence gives no indication whether *all* important components — between fifteen and twenty-five for a clinical department — are to be evaluated during a particular time period or in a set frequency. The determination of performance standards for each component should be attainable, but the apparent equation of criteria with indicators will cause real confusion. The collection of data to determine performance suggests routine monitoring and pays scant attention to different types of data and standards.

Chapter 4 of this book deals with performance assessment, and there we review four different sources of data or viewpoints on clinical and service performance.

Response

Clause #6.   *Action is taken when problems are identified.*
   6.1   *The plan of action for each problem outlines. . . [alternatives and most appropriate action, time required and person responsible]. . . .*

Clause #7.   *Actions are followed up within a specified timeframe to ensure that they are effective.*
   7.1   *To assess the effectiveness, evaluation methods are utilized. These methods may include: re-audit, re-survey, ongoing review of quality indicators.*

There has always been a strong imperative within QA to take responsibility for, and respond appropriately to, data discovered through quality assurance. This probably reached its height during the days when QA was defined as problem solving, i.e., the 1983 *Standards* in Canada. The rule today is for departments to follow up the analysis of data with the staff's evaluation of its findings. Then management must take appropriate action, as follows:

- The department may approve of its findings and choose to report them without more ado.

- It may approve them in general, but note and act upon an opportunity for minor improvement. Reporting and improvement will be concurrent. Or,

- It may be severely dissatisfied with its findings, in which case it will develop a plan of action, as suggested in the *Standard*, outlining "alternative actions to solve the problem, the most appropriate action, the time required to implement the action, the person(s) responsible for taking action" (Clause 6.1).

In this eventuality, the action plan takes the place of the QA report, in communicating results to the senior echelons in the facility. Later it is expected that the department will return to the topic or performance and reaudit; if satisfied, it will report, and continue to monitor to ensure the maintenance of the new level of performance.

2.4
The
Effectiveness
of QA

The Reality of Improvement

Although the *Standards* are simple and direct, there are two problems with their observance: the reality of improvement and the quality of reporting. There has long been doubt about the extent to which QA has been successful in changing physician behaviour. Wyszewianski[6] says that the problem is broader than that. Although there is the formula:

$$\text{Quality Assurance} = \text{Quality assessment (measurement)} + \text{Quality improvement and control (action)},[7]$$

in fact all QA's efforts and expertise have gone into measurement and not action. The new advocates of CQI agree. In fact, they justify QA's ineffectiveness in bringing about improvement by pointing to the fact that management expects the department to solve its own QA problems without showing it how or providing resources or support. In CQI the responsibility for change and the enthusiasm for improvement begin at the top of the organization, and CQI provides a tool kit of data analysis and display techniques for those engaged in improvement projects.

Most people in quality assurance would agree that Wyszewianski and the CQI advocates have indeed revealed QA's Achilles' heel.

The Quality of Reporting

After suggesting that QA does not cut the mustard as an action strategy, it may seem anticlimactic to discuss the quality of the paperwork. There are two points to be raised in defence of QA. The first is the question: Where would we be without QA? Without its continuous monitoring and daily focus on quality of performance, it is probable that performance would be much less reliable and standards far less strict. I am reminded of the experience of having carried out a preaccreditation survey of a long-term care facility that had voluntarily stepped out of the hospital accreditation program. What I and my physician colleague discovered was a facility that had failed to keep up, to bring on board the essential practices that had been introduced into the field since their last survey some eight years earlier. The hospital had become a backwater. The experience gave me a new respect for the effectiveness of the accreditation program in inducing change. It is probable that continuous QA is highly influential in similarly maintaining momentum and in keeping quality high on the agenda of practitioners.

The second point is that for all QA's supposed impotence, knowledge of what is needed is the essential first step in seeking to achieve that goal. The recognition of industry benchmarks, the review of the data and response of others will motivate practitioners to want to do better.

Since publishing *Hospital-wide Quality Assurance* in 1987, I have felt compelled to address the need for better focussed and more worthwhile QA reports and set limits on the volume and frequency of QA reporting. In the first of two papers, "Evaluating QA Reports: Five Standards,"[8] I stressed the importance of aiming QA efforts and reports at worthwhile and potentially valuable topics. The five standards address the choice of topic, method of assessment, appropriateness of conclusions, follow-up action and comprehensibility of the report. The second article, "Reporting Quality: Reasonable Demands of the QA Program,"[9] returned to the crusade against insignificant audits and fragmented appraisals and proposed the "five Cs" of QA reports: they must be continuous, comprehensive, comparable, of consequence, and concise. The method recommended whereby QA reporting could meet these five criteria is the QA Calendar described in Chapter 4.

2.5
Trustees and Quality of Care

Receiving QA reports and understanding their implications have been difficult assignments for lay trustees. The task can be made less daunting if the reporters, executives and medical leaders understand that there are five questions that lay trustees should ask and be given answers to:

- What do our patients/clients think about the quality of care?

- What do the experts (i.e., external inspection reports) say about it?

- What do the hospital's outcomes (indicators) look like?

- How are our clinicians and others monitoring or assuring quality of care? and

- What do their reviews or audits tell them and us?

Exhibit 2.2
Bibliography: Trustees and Quality Assurance

Bader, Barry S. (1991). *Informing the Board about Quality* and *Informing the Board about Medical Staff Credentialling and Development.* (Two books.) Rockville, MD: Bader & Associates.

Berwick, Donald M., Godfrey, A. Blanton, and Roessner, Jane (1990). *Curing Health Care: A Report on the National Demonstration Project on Quality Improvement in Health Care. New Strategies for Quality Improvement.* San Francisco: Jossey-Bass.

Goldfield, N. and Nash, D.B., eds. (1989). *Providing Quality Care: The Challenge to Physicians.* Philadelphia: American College of Physicians.

Orlikoff, J.E. and Totten, M.K. (1991). *The Board's Role in Quality Care: A Practical Guide for Hospital Trustees.* Chicago: American Hospital Publishing.

Walton, M. (1986). *The Deming Management Method.* New York: Putnam.

Williams, K.J. and Donnelly, P.R. (1987). *Medical Care Quality and the Public Trust.* Ottawa: Canadian Hospital Association.

Wilson, C.R.M. (1987). *Hospital-wide Quality Assurance: Models for implementation and Development.* Toronto: W.B. Saunders, Chapter VIII.

Wilson, C.R.M. (1991). *New on Board: Essentials of Governance for Hospital Trustees.* Ottawa: Canadian Hospital Association, Chapter 7.

If boards insist that their QA committees — however they are titled — are composed predominantly of lay trustees, and those committees insist that these questions be asked at each meeting, it is likely that lay language will be spoken and that information will gain ascendency over data. Few situations are more discouraging than seeing trustees bombarded with answers to questions they have not asked, or reading the bewilderment on their faces as they try to grapple with clinical or technical information. Exhibit 2.2 provides a short list of material on quality written for trustees or generalists.

2.6
Conclusion: In Defence of Models

This chapter has introduced the PIER model; Chapter 4 will discuss PAIX. If readers turn to the chapters on medical QA they will meet the Four-Legged Table. The risk management section explores CRIPPLE (the Risk Heptagon), while the essentials of CQI are remembered through the word PROCESS. No, this is not Sesame Street or Children's Hour; both models and mnemonics (memory aids) are of practical importance in implementing quality assurance. If a facility's QA program is to be consistent, it needs to be based on the same amalgam of essential activities, constructs and values. This amalgam is the model. The mnemonics are an ideal vehicle for quality assurance for three reasons: First, models distill a mass of discussion, theory, structures and practices into one formula, a single list of what needs to be known or done and in what order. Second, they commit the management of quality assurance into the hands of department heads or head nurses and their staff. These people need practical, actionable precepts, not a *smorgasbord* of concepts and possibilities. Third, both they and I need the formula in a memorable form. I need a memory aid in order to teach a wide variety of audiences, in various situations — from one-on-one to seventy or more people sitting in a fixed-seat auditorium — and always without notes. Managers too find it helpful to receive their marching orders in a secure container. Models and memory aids increase the likelihood that all a facility's department heads will do QA the same way when each one returns to his or her department or nursing unit.

Last week I was at a thirty-four bed, acute-care hospital in Northwestern Ontario. All of its department heads and head nurses were working supervisors. They needed their QA tasks to be intelligible, practical and essential, i.e. the minimum theory necessary for basic assurance. In forty-eight hours I had to take this management team from a definition of the 1992 QA *Standard,* through audit and indicators, to the development of a QA Calendar for each department. This week I must do the same for a military hospital. After reviewing what was available, they have chosen the PIER model and have given themselves six weeks to install and operate it effectively. PIER may have appealed to this facility because health care personnel in the armed services rotate through the hospital, and a simple and memorable system may survive the changes in staff better than one that depends on resident QA specialists.

However, I am aware, as the reader will be, that the value of the model is not in its simplicity — it can simply be wrong — but in the experience and scholarship from which its precepts are drawn. All the models and recommendations in this book meet the three tests of necessity (i.e., you need to do it), practicality (it works), and literature support (clinicians and/or academics have proposed or endorsed the concepts). Of course, not all academics, practitioners or clinicians will endorse any one model, because in the nature of things models reflect the choices of their developer. Some of my biases are evident already: for example, *against* management content, *for* indicators; *against* structure, *for* outcome. My choices have been made with the intention of providing practitioners with simple directions to an economical and tightly focussed QA program. As well as debriding the area of dead and useless material, the models are intended to propose new patient-centred and service-based activities that should appeal to clinicians and service providers. Quality assurance takes its vitality and interest from the work it examines.

References

1. All quotations from the *Standards* given in this chapter, unless otherwise indicated, come from the "Quality Assurance Standard Area" (VII for patient care departments, VI for support services). In this and most cases they are reproduced with the clause number that occurs within the Standard Area.

2. Ontario Hospital Association and Ontario Medical Association (1990). *OHA, OMA Prototype Hospital By-laws*. Toronto: OHA, pp. 60 and 63.

3. Wilson, C.R.M. (1987). *Hospital-wide Quality Assurance*. Toronto: W.B. Saunders, pp.18-21, 81-103, 126-127.

4. *Ibid*.

5. 1991 *Standards*. Quality Assurance Standard Area: Clauses 4 and 5.

6. Wyszewianski, L. (1988). The emphasis on measurement in quality assurance: Reasons and implications. *Inquiry* 25(Winter):424-436.

7. *Ibid*., p. 425.

8. Wilson, C.R.M. (1988). Evaluating QA reports: Five standards. *Quality Assurance Quarterly (CAQAP)* 5(2 [Feb.]):3-6.

9. Wilson, C.R.M. (1989). Reporting quality: Reasonable demands of the QA program. *Quality Assurance Quarterly (CAQAP)* 7(11 [Nov.]):13-16.

3

Performance Indicators

3.1
An Open Letter to
the Council

In September 1989 an event occurred in Canadian health care politics that was highly unusual. Five national bodies, four of whom appointed members to seats on its board, wrote an open letter to the Canadian Council on Health Facilities Accreditation (CCHFA). In their *Joint Statement*, the Canadian Hospital Association (CHA), Canadian Long Term Care Association, Canadian Medical Association, Canadian Nurses Association and Canadian Standards Association demanded the promotion and use of outcome-oriented indicators in quality assurance. The preamble to the *Joint Statement* and its final section ("Recommendations for Action") are here reproduced in their entirety:

Preamble

The co-sponsors are committed to promote quality assurance in health care facilities that is systematic, meaningful, integrated into the management of care/service delivery and linked with other ongoing evaluative activities.

Different settings and circumstances determine the approach selected to assess quality. To date, quality assurance in health care facilities has tended to concentrate on those characteristics that are believed to reflect quality in the setting and process of care or service. The co-sponsors are committed to build into quality assurance the capacity to also focus on the results or outcome of care or service for the consumer. The co-sponsors believe that outcome-oriented indicators of quality, applied in the context of meaningful quality assurance programmes, are an efficient way to accomplish this.

The co-sponsors recognize that it is often difficult to clearly establish a cause/effect relationship between care or service and subsequent results, to accurately measure results and to attribute results to antecedent care or service; however, an outcome orientation in the selection of indicators focuses attention on managing care or service to increase the probability of achieving desired results and reducing the probability of undesired results. . . .

Recommendations for Action

The co-sponsors pledge their support and assistance in ongoing efforts to develop outcome-oriented indicators.

The following recommendations for action are intended to act as reference points for the co-sponsors as they work to support and strengthen current efforts to manage quality in health care facilities.

1. The co-sponsors recommend that the Canadian Council on Health Facilities Accreditation (CCHFA) develop and endorse a definition of quality health care/service based on the following:

    'Quality' health care/service is care or service with characteristics that meet specified requirements and, given the current state of knowledge and available

> *resources, fulfill reasonable expectations for maximizing benefits and minimizing risks to the health and well-being of the consumer.*
>
> 2. *The co-sponsors recommend timely action by CCHFA in collaboration with relevant national health organizations and other accrediting bodies to develop and validate relevant, practical, outcome-oriented indicators of quality for high-volume, high-risk, problem-prone areas of care/service in Canadian health care facilities.*
>
> *Efforts should be founded on grassroots involvement in developing indicators. Prior to formal endorsement of indicators by national health organizations and/or accrediting bodies, field trials are needed to critically assess whether use of these indicators actually contributes to quality improvement.*
>
> *Furthermore, ongoing critical review of established indicators is required to ensure that indicators in use in the field are current and relevant.*[1]

In the preamble, the sponsors advocated the use of outcome-oriented indicators for three reasons: the efficiency of indicators in focussing on outcome, their effectiveness in influencing results, and their usefulness in decision making.

The sponsors' recommendations for action demonstrate their own commitment to quality assurance and to the development and widest possible use of outcome indicators. The early drafts of the 1991 *Standards* gave the hope that CCHFA was going to follow the lead of its national members. Unfortunately, in my view, the Council ultimately chose to endorse neither the use of indicators, nor an outcome focus in the 1991 *Standards*. It did, however, continue with the Outcomes Measurement Project it had initiated in October 1989. We will need to revisit this decision below, when we look at global or facility outcomes/indicators. But first we need to define what is meant by an indicator, to look at how indicators are or can be used, and to provide some means by which departments can generate indicators appropriate to their functions.

3.2 Defining Indicators

In September 1990 the Joint Commission on the Accreditation of Healthcare Organizations (JCAHO) brought a one-day in-house program to Kingston General Hospital, led by Robert J. Marder, MD and C. Irving Meeker, MD. With due acknowledgement to the JCAHO and its material,[2] we can make the following summary statements about performance indicators:

1. An indicator is a quantity that tells us something about quality. It is always a number.

2. Indicators are signs, flags or signals. They are a quick balance, a look at the bottom line, a sign of the times.

3. Indicators are not infallible. Their meaning is not clear until they are investigated.

4. Indicators are of two kinds:
   - *sentinel events,* i.e., single, highly significant events such as a death, an automobile accident, a fire, or a lawsuit, which require immediate investigation; or
   - *rate-based indicators,* such as (rates of) infections, accidents, Caesarean sections, film retakes, that will be monitored regularly and investigated periodically and when they vary significantly from their mean or norm.[3]

5. Indicators can be positive or negative. They are more than Elinson's "five Ds" (death, disease, disability, discomfort and dissatisfaction).[4] (See Exhibit 3.2 for non-clinical examples.)

6. Indicators can be defined in five dimensions (see Exhibit 3.1).

Exhibit 3.1
Indicator Profile: Five Dimensions

Process	or	Outcome
Sentinel event	and/or	Rate-based
Effectiveness	and/or	Appropriateness
Adverse event	or	Desirable event
Practitioner-focussed	or	System-focussed

— Joint Commission on Accreditation of Healthcare Organizations (JCAHO), Kingston General Hospital Custom Program, September 1990; and JCAHO (1990), *Primer on Indicator Developement and Application,* pp. 8-9.

Unfortunately, not everyone uses the term "indicator" in the same way; in fact, both of the Canadian authorities quoted offer other definitions. In their *Joint Statement,* the CHA *et al.* give this definition:

An outcome-oriented indicator is a defined, measurable aspect of a characteristic of care or service that can be attributed to antecedent care or service. For example, the number of consumer complaints is an indicator of consumer satisfaction, a reflection of quality in the outcome of care; the degree of symptom remission is an indicator of achievement of expected/desired benefits, a reflection of quality in the outcome of care.[5]

Earlier, in the preamble quoted above, the authors had acknowledged the difficulties in "establish[ing] a cause/effect relationship between care or service and subsequent results" and attributing "results to antecedent care". They illustrate these difficulties well in one example used in their definition. Patient complaints/satisfaction are a direct function not of the quality of care but the expectations of the patient.[6]
    The second definition that deserves attention is that of

the CCHFA, which uses the terms "indicator" and "criterion" interchangeably:

> *Criteria. . . [are] measurable indicators of the achievement of a standard; defined measurable variables relating to the structure, process or outcome of important aspects of care for which data are collected in the monitoring and evaluation process.*[7]

There is a contrast of magnitude between the Council's indicators/criteria, which define the components of a standard, and the sentinel events and rate-based indicators I mentioned earlier. A good indicator should wave its own flag. The Council's are a large handful of straws in the wind.

In my definition I have leaned heavily on material presented in the JCAHO program. The JCAHO's official publication on the subject is *Primer on Indicator Development and Application: Measuring Quality in Health Care* (1990).[8] In fairness to JCAHO and its *Primer,* it should be noted that the Joint Commission advocates much stricter standards in indicator development and testing than I consider practical or :ssary to the assurance of health care quality in Canada.

3.3
Living in an
Indicator Society

On two occasions last fall I had the same experience. I was sitting in the airport in Ottawa awaiting the call to board my flight home to Toronto. Having taught indicators all day, I was glad to sit still and relax and forget all about indicators and quality assurance, and reach for the novel I was carrying. But it was not to be. Staring at me was an electronic board that carried, in Canada's two official languages, sports scores and headlines and data from the financial markets. And doing her rounds of business travellers was a university student distributing *The Globe & Mail Afternoon Report on Business,* a single-sheet hand-out replete with the local, national and international — you guessed it — indicators for that day, Thursday, 24 October 1991. Inescapably, we live in an indicator society!

"What do the following have in common?" I ask participants in my indicator workshops. "The Dow Jones Industrial Average, the birth rate, traffic fatalities per year, number of housing starts, a patient's vital signs, RBIs, ERAs and stolen bases?"

Audiences give me some of the following answers: "They are all numbers." "They go up and down." "They are probably all commonly used — but only by people in a particular field." "They are not 'sure things', i.e., they can give false positives and false negatives." "They are used both to tell you what is going on and for predicting what is likely to happen."

With minimal response to the audience's comments, I will then show them a slide on which are listed the names of a dozen or so hospital departments and ask them to suggest an indicator for each of them. Their most common responses are shown in Exhibit 3.2.

I intend by these two exercises to demonstrate two features of indicators: First, that indicators are part of the patterns of everyday thought and speech in North America. We think and talk in comparative, perhaps even competitive terms. There are indicators in every newscast, on the front page of every newspaper. Each *cause célèbre* develops its own, whether it be the Gulf War or an oil spill in Alaska. Sports is replete with them. I have a Toronto Blue Jays playbook that on one page lists twenty-two indicators, and that is just for batting. Pitching accounts for another fourteen!

Second, indicators are highly accessible in health care. Professionals have little difficulty in identifying important indicators for the major functions of their facility. If we expect department heads to use performance indicators naturally, we must demystify them or not allow them to become "scientized", i.e., a special possession of the experts.

Exhibit 3.2
Indicators Suggested by Audiences for Major Hospital Departments

Finance	Amount of hospital's deficit
Surgery	Postsurgical infection rate
Obstetrics	Number of live births
Food Services	Patient satisfaction scores
Hospital Safety	Number of lost-time injuries
Emergency	Waiting time
Radiology	Film retake rate
Plant & Engineering	Breakdowns
Payroll	Number of manual cheques
Nursing	Medication incidents

3.4
Identifying Indicators: Four Routes

A new manager of Human Resources (HR) asked for help in the development of indicators for her function. Having worked for four years in a human resources directorate, I tried to recall what were the key issues my colleagues dealt with. I came up with three: employee turnover rate; number of grievances; and number of lost-time injuries per X thousand paid hours.

All of these statistics are important in personnel; none of them is directly attributable to the human resources function. These are global or facility-wide indicators. Then I ran my eyes down the list of principal functions I had hypothesized for the HR department: recruitment; salary and benefit administration; labour relations; HR policy administration; and personal records. Again reaching back fifteen years, I suggested, in this order:

- Separations within a year

- Compensation incidents

- Grievances

- Sickness and absence rates

- Performance appraisal completion.

I have recounted this experience because the first place to start discovering indicators is with a plain piece of paper and your own experience. Indicators can also be found or developed in at least three other ways: by prescription, through the audit process, and by activity mapping. As only the last is specifically described in the literature, it is worthwhile to explain each method in turn.

From Experience

Imagine the following scenario: You have an opportunity to assess a department similar to your own in another facility. Your time there will be very limited. What will you look at or ask about? What indications will you use to tell you how well it is operating?

If the reader were to go through this exercise — as have hundreds of managers in workshops with me in 1991 — he or she would probably list many indicators of structure: the size, resources and staffing of the department; process indicators, such as the scope of the department's operation, the range of its products or services. Beyond these should lie some answers to the question of how well the department is doing. These answers may relate to the facility as client

Exhibit 3.3
Some Common Departmental Indicators

Length of stay (Nursing)

Patient satisfaction scores (various)

Complaints (various)

Waiting lists (Rehabilitation)

Cancellations (Surgery)

Dispensing errors (Pharmacy)

Employee turnover rate (Nursing)

Referrals (Pastoral Care)

(productivity and solvency), but others will deal with either the *content,* i.e., the outcome of the service or production, or its *delivery* as perceived by its clients. These are the key or leading indicators that department heads need to find. They tend to be well recognized within the field and readily explicable to those outside. The suggestions given by managers in Exhibit 3.3 would be good examples.

By Prescription

The second method is taken from the text of the QA *Standard,* Clauses 4 and 5. In a series of steps, they refer to:

- principal functions,

- their important components,

- setting standards of performance for these components, and

- identifying the test or indicator that will show whether the department performed to its expectations or not.

Two examples will help; they are given in Exhibit 3.4. The first deals with a principal function of Materiel Management: the purchasing of non-stock items. The second, in Nursing, is concerned with the planning of care.

Exhibit 3.4
Establishing Indicators by Prescription

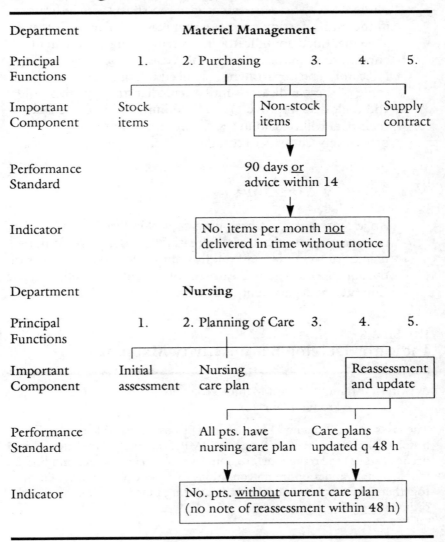

Department	**Materiel Management**				
Principal Functions	1.	2. Purchasing	3.	4.	5.
Important Component	Stock items		Non-stock items		Supply contract
Performance Standard			90 days or advice within 14		
Indicator			No. items per month not delivered in time without notice		

Department	**Nursing**				
Principal Functions	1.	2. Planning of Care	3.	4.	5.
Important Component	Initial assessment	Nursing care plan		Reassessment and update	
Performance Standard		All pts. have nursing care plan	Care plans updated q 48 h		
Indicator		No. pts. without current care plan (no note of reassessment within 48 h)			

Through the Audit Process

A full description of the audit process is provided in Chapter 4. When audit teams come to summarize their findings, more often than not they will do so in indicator terms: percentage of cases not followed up, percentage of antibiotics used without clinical justification, number of outliers, etc. The department may return to these indicators in the future for any one of several reasons. The audit may have identified an indicator important enough and patent enough to monitor on a monthly basis — a leading or risk indicator. The department may need to continue to monitor some of these indicators until a remedial strategy takes hold and their data improve. At a minimum, the indicators and their data will remain in the file in case or until the department chooses to reaudit the same or an allied topic.

Via Activity Mapping

An accepted way of developing clinical indicators is to construct a flow chart of the treatment process, or a criteria map.[9] For example, staff might want to develop indicators of the appropriateness of treatment of patients presenting in the Emergency department with acute chest pain. The flow

Exhibit 3.5
Indicator Development: Activity Mapping

Activity: Arranging Board Mentor Programs
Role: Program Director

The tasks of the Program Director are (1) to make available to member hospitals the Board Mentor Program (BMP) which OHA operates under licence and (2) to arrange the program so that hospital boards and board mentors meet under optimum conditions to experience the program together. The first is an advertising/marketing function, the second a co-ordinating one.

Activity	Possible Indicators
1. Program Director (PD) advertises availability of program to member hospitals (H) by means of information meetings, appearances of mentors, mailings and literature.	No. inquiries, applications, programs completed p.a.
2. PD provides answers to H questions, including when to have and not to have program, and who should attend.	The wrong people can attend — too few trustees, too many executives.
3. PD checks the H's application to clarify appropriate dates, program duration and lead time.	CEO may not get all the materials H needs.
4. PD sends H enough copies of the program materials and a list of mentors (M), whom H should rank-order.	Because of other M commitments, H may not get its choice of M.
5. When H has indicated its preferences, PD approaches mentors in turn to engage their services.	M may not receive all they need from OHA or materials from H.
6. PD sends to M a kit of material which M will need in acting as board mentor.	Not all board members complete SAS or attend.
7. H has to distribute self-assessment surveys (SAS) for completion by all board members and CEO, collect them, collate the data and send collation and SAS to M 7 days prior to retreat.	Collation and SAS can reach M late.
8. Participants evaluate BMP retreat and mentor.	More than 75% indicates an Excellent rating.

Indicators Chosen

1. No. programs completed per year (Item 1).

2. No. complications occurring per program (Items 2-7).

3. Numerical rating on participant evaluations at the conclusion of the retreat (Item 8).

chart would begin with the patient presenting in Emergency:
Was he or she seen by a nurse for triage? Yes/No.

If Yes, did the nurse recognize the possibility of the acute
nature of P's condition? Yes/No.

In the flow chart, each Yes shows that the recommended
clinical process is on track. Each No represents a deviation,
an unnecessary detour in P's progress towards appropriate
diagnosis and, hopefully, effective care — and thus a negative
indicator.

I have, for demonstration purposes, applied this activity
mapping to a non-clinical function for which I once had
responsibility: managing the Ontario Hospital Association's
Board Mentor Program (Exhibit 3.5). It yielded both
positive indicators (e.g., the number of programs purchased
per year) and negative indicators — deviations from the
process that might complicate or threaten the success of the
program for the mentors or the program's client facilities
(wrong people, inappropriate setting, failure to deliver
needed materials in time, or failure to gain co-operation of
the CEO).

3.5
Putting Indicators
in Context

"How would you feel if I told you that at 11:00 the Dow
Jones Industrial Average had hit the 1500 mark?"

The nurse looked at me as if I were talking a foreign
language — which of course I was — and replied, "It
wouldn't bother me!"

Indicators viewed without a structured numerical
context are mute; without one or more comparators, they
say nothing.

The room cleaning score for housekeeping was 78% for
October: an indicator. Radiology's retake rate for the same

month was 3.2%: another indicator. On inspection by the Public Health Department, Food Services was served with two orders: yet another indicator. But what do they mean?

The orders issued by the Public Health Department were sentinel events; their content is more important than their number. They have to be reviewed on their merits, and of course addressed. But how about the scores from Housekeeping and Radiology? Like the Dow Jones Industrial average, they must be reviewed in their numerical context.

There are several dimensions that go to make up the numerical context of an indicator. The following features should be illustrated on an indicator run or trend chart, which is the recommended vehicle to use in reporting an indicator.

1. *Actual scores* for each of the previous three months and the same month last year.

2. *The historical range.* High and low scores for this year and the previous year, and the mean score for last year.

3. *An industry benchmark.* Each year the department should look to its professional society or hospital peer group for a benchmark or industrial standard of performance. This should be based on actuals achieved and not an ideal score.

In addition to these figures, the department may need to specify the following:

4. *A fixed standard.* If their activity has a fixed 0-or-100% standard, such as in the administration of medications, surgical cancellations or complications, this standard should be registered. Or:

5. *A departmental/program target.* In the absence of a legislated or fixed standard, the department may be free to set its own target, i.e., the performance level with which it would be pleased. It may also need to set

6. *A minimal acceptable score* to denote a performance level with which it would be displeased.

7. Between Items 5 and 6 — the target and the minimum
    — the department should set its *threshold for action,* i.e.,
    the point at which the department would begin to take
    action to halt a downward trend in its performance.

These features are illustrated in Exhibit 3.6.

Exhibit 3.6
Indicators in Their Numerical Context

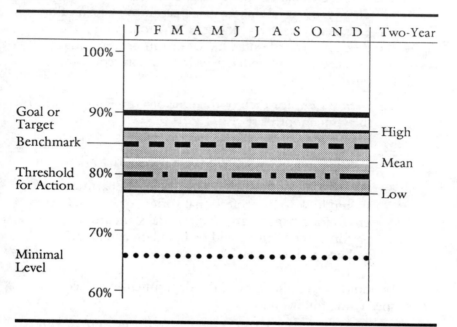

It is worth noting that all these benchmarks, goals,
targets, scores and thresholds are standards, i.e., "levels of
excellence or quality"[10], a term we have chosen to use
sparingly. One of the reasons that the word "standard" is so
misunderstood is that it is a generic term. In the QA
literature it is used almost exclusively as a desirable score,
level or achievement, whereas in common parlance it can be
negative (a poor standard of living) or positive (a high
standard of care).

3.6 Using Indicators in the QA Program

The availability of four methods of indicator development carries the probability that a manager could end up with hundreds of indicators, many of them of questionable or no value. Thus, the first task is to categorize them by use. The second is to recognize that there are practical limits to the number of indicators that can be monitored before they all become undiscriminated data. The third task is to find some criteria that will help managers choose between available indicators.

Priorities

It is useful to sort indicators into four categories or priorities for use. These are:

Priority 1: Risk indicators
Always important; must be recorded and reviewed at earliest opportunity: patient deaths, fires, crime, wound infections.

Priority 2: Leading or key indicators
Always important; highly sensitive and indicative of operation of department/facility: number of grievances, length of stay, surgical cancellations, sickness/absence rates. Should be kept and plotted on a monthly basis.

Priority 3: Descriptive indicators
Useful. These indicators become important when their values change significantly, but are not important enough to report regularly or are too expensive to generate except when specifically relevant.

Priority 0: Dispensible data

Of questionable or no value. All sorts of figures can be
generated that may be useful to management and relevant in
the context of an audit or other inquiry but tell the
department nothing important as stand-alone data — the
test of an indicator. Do not collect or report.

From the description of these categories it will be clear
what managers should do with Priority 1 and 0 indicators.
They will report immediately and monitor monthly risk
indicators; they will discard 0 indicators as unnecessary and
inarticulate constructs.

Setting Limits

It is difficult to be as categorical about key indicators.
Technical departments have multitudes of available
indicators. Their professionals also have a greater facility for
handling quantities of numerical data. In Engineering and
Plant Maintenance they may be monitoring fifteen to twenty
indicators each hour and looking at summary data on them
and others on a daily basis. In Laboratories they will maintain
a run chart on each piece of diagnostic equipment and on
the quality control samples they test daily or more frequently.
For departments such as these, the corrective might be to
insist that to be a key or leading indicator the quantity
should be the one, chosen from many, that is both the best
indicator of quality of performance and is easily explicable to
the lay mind — in management and on the board.
The ideal is for line departments to arrive at the point
where they have a risk or key indicator for each of their
principal functions, and for their total number not to exceed
twelve. For many, six to eight will be a more manageable
number. I am aware that other people use many more
indicators, and use them differently from the way I describe.
For example, the department of Surgery at the Hospital for
Sick Children lists a total of thirty indicators: twenty

monitored per month, eight per quarter and two semi-annually.[11] The vast majority of these will be, according to our classification, descriptive indicators.

We have advised smaller and less automated departments to focus on risk and key indicators, to monitor them monthly and — once a year — to revisit each monthly indicator or group of related indicators and analyze the data behind the figures to look for reasons and trends. This revisit and analysis will occur as a scheduled entry in the department's QA Calendar (Chapter 4).

Descriptive indicators are not reported on a monthly basis unless they are useful data on implementing a strategy to improve unsatisfactory performance. However, reference may be made to them when the data behind a related key indicator are being reviewed in the annual revisit.

Making Choices

It is easy to lose sight of the fact that we are looking for the indicator that tells it all: the smoking gun, the bottom line, rather than a flurry of circumstantial evidence. Sickness and absence rates have proved to be the best barometer of an employee group's morale. In a long-term care facility, the number of decubitus ulcers is one of the best indicators of the quality of nursing care. The search is for the few, sensitive, and important figures that will enable us and others to take a quick read of current performance. When faced with an overabundance of possible indicators there are two strategies available to department heads: they should resort to some clear criteria in making choices; and they can look at the possibility of bunching indicators to increase their power. A good indicator should meet the following criteria in the order listed:

1. *Significance.* The data must be of real importance to the reporting department, whether or not they are directly attributable to its efforts. Thus, the postsurgical infection rate is a necessary indicator for a surgical nursing unit.

2. *Validity.* The data must measure accurately what they are supposed to reflect. Thus, charting should not be allowed to stand for care, or numbers of patient complaints for patient satisfaction. It is worth noting that "medication incidents", one of the most popular risk indicators, is a highly questionable statistic because it is based on self-reported data.

3. *Availability of data.* Indicators are intended to be a highly efficient method of monitoring performance by means of available data. If departments have to dig for or calculate the data, they should think about downgrading the indicator from key to descriptive, and review and report it on an irregular basis.

4. *Sensitivity.* An indicator must indicate. That is, it must be sensitive to changes in the performance from which its data are derived. In addition, the changes it registers should in the main be attributable to changes in quality of performance, rather than reflect a variety of other variables.

5. *Professional respect.* While local indicators will often be most sensitive to the work of the department, there is merit in using indicators that are widely used in the department's own field or by its lead profession. Departments that do not use popular indicators are asked why. Trustees and senior management want their departments to use standards that allow comparisons with others.

Bunching: Two Examples

A cardiopulmonary unit (CPU) generated for its three clinical functions eight, six and two indicators. On further analysis, a consultant recommended that the sixteen be collapsed into six, more generic, indicators. After each is listed, the number of proposed indicators were combined into the new definition:

1. Risk   Patient adverse occurrences (2)

2. Risk   Mechanical malfunction/breakdown of
               CPU equipment (1)

3. Leading   Complaints and commendations per
               quarter, patient and MD (5)

4. Leading   Tests cancelled/repeated per month
               divided by total tests scheduled (4)

5. Leading   Failure to meet department's standards for
               timeliness of attention (4)

6. Descriptive LOS by category (1)

In a facility for the developmentally challenged,
Vocational Services had to:

- arrange service contracts with commercial companies, so
  as to

- provide work opportunities for residents,

- assess the residents' needs, interests and abilities, and

- train and supervise them in the work assignments.

In developing an indicator for these important components
of two principal functions, the department rejected:

- The number and volume of commercial contracts. The
  important feature of the contracts was their ability to
  provide work within the capability and the interest/
  attention span of the residents, because they could walk
  off the job whenever they chose.

- The monthly earnings from these contracts, because
  work experience was the purpose, not offset revenue.

- Total resident attendance, because each resident had his
  or her own recommended duration of work experience.

The department instead chose "the percent of the
residents per week who met or exceeded the number of hours
of work experience recommended for them." This indicator

would be sensitive to the volume and appropriateness of work contracts secured, the tasking of the work, the individual assignment of residents to appropriate tasks, and the training and supervision provided for them. The data needed (number of residents on work experience, recommended duration, and attendance) all came off one sheet of paper: the attendance record.

Exhibits 3.7 through 3.12 provide examples of some indicators from Nursing, Pharmacy, a therapy (Physiotherapy), mental health/ counselling (Social Work), a science (Food Services) and a staff department (Human Resources).

Exhibit 3.7
Principal Functions and Performance Indicators

Department: Nursing, Acute Care

Principal Functions	*Performance Indicators*
1. Assessment and planning of care	Failure to assess correctly
2. Intervention/treatment	Medical incidents Infection rate
3. Personal care	Complaints from family
4. Pt. education	Complaints and commendations Discharges without appropriate instructions
5. Provision of safe and comfortable environment	Pt. incidents (falls, wandering, etc.) No. discrepancies on safety inspections

Note: Principal functions are given to show the range of work carried out by department. Indicators may or may not fit with one or more functions.

Exhibit 3.8
Principal Functions and Performance Indicators

Department: Pharmacy

Principal Functions

Performance Indicators

1. Purchasing and inventory
    control incl. formulary

Inventory turnover rate
Size of formulary
% of budget spent on anti-infectives

2. Dispensing/ manufacturing

3. Distribution

4. Clinical pharmacy

% of pharmacist advice accepted by
physicians

5. Drug information

6. Pt. education

% of pts. counselled by pharmacy

Note: Principal functions are given to show the range of work carried out
by department. Indicators may or may not fit with one or more functions.

— *Dimensions 66* (Nov. 1989):13-15.

Exhibit 3.9
Principal Functions and Performance Indicators

Department: Physiotherapy

Principal Functions	*Performance Indicators*
1. Assessment	
2. Treatment/in-patient	Lengths of time on waiting list % pts. achieving treatment goals on time
3. Treatment/out-patient	OP cancellation rate
4. Pt./family education	
5. Communication and charting	% appropriate/inappropriate referrals
6. Health Education/Students, other staff	% time on direct vs. indirect care

Note: Principal functions are given to show the range of work carried out by department. Indicators may or may not fit with one or more functions.

— *Dimensions 67* (Feb. 1990):15-17.

Exhibit 3.10
Principal Functions and Performance Indicators

Department: Social Work Services

Principal Functions	*Performance Indicators*
1. Assessment/intake	% pts. seen by Social Work Accuracy of assessment
2. Crisis intervention	
3. Pt./family counselling	% of planned results not achieved Timeliness of service Readmissions with social complications
4. Community liaison/referral	Discharge delays Pt./family involved in discharge plan % pts. seen after discharge
5. Communication and charting	No. Social Work pts. discharged without SW knowledge

Note: Principal functions are given to show the range of work carried out by department. Indicators may or may not fit with one or more functions.

—Vourlekis, B.S. (1990). The field's evaluation of proposed clinical indicators for social work sciences in the acute-care hospital. *Health and Social Work* 15(3 [Aug.]):197-206.

Exhibit 3.11
Principal Functions and Performance Indicators

Department: Food Services*

Principal Functions	*Performance Indicators*
1. Purchasing/inventory control	Overage/shortage per month Food waste ($) per mo.
2. Menu planning/food preparation	Tray audit scores
3. Patient food service	Pt. food survey score No. trays returned untouched
4. Cafeteria/special catering	Cafeteria survey scores Gross take ($) per month
5. Sanitation	No. discrepancies on Public Health inspection No. employee incidents

* Not incl.: Therapeutic Nutrition

Note: Principal functions are given to show the range of work carried out by department. Indicators may or may not fit with one or more functions.

Exhibit 3.12
Principal Functions and Performance Indicators

Department: Human Resources

Principal Functions	*Performance Indicators*
1. Recruitment	Staff vacancy rate
	Separations within 1 year
2. Salary administration, incl. benefits	Compensation incidents
3. Personnel records	Performance appraisal completions
4. Labour relations	No. grievances
	Sickness and absence rates
5. Policy administration (human rights, etc.)	Employee turnover
6. Staff counselling	

Note: Principal functions are given to show the range of work carried out by department. Indicators may or may not fit with one or more functions.

3.7
Global Indicators

Wyszewianski writes:

> *Because the delivery of health services is complex and has multiple goals — of which postponing death is but one — no single measure is apt to capture overall quality. Still everyone would like to have a universal "quality meter" that readily generates for each provider an overall score that is both valid and meaningful.*[12]

Exhibit 3.13
MHA Quality Indicator Project

List of Indicators

1. Hospital-acquired infections
2. Surgical wound infections
3. In-patient mortality
4. Neonatal mortality
5. Perioperative mortality
6. Caesarean sections
7. Unplanned readmissions
8. Unplanned admissions following ambulatory surgery
9. Unplanned returns to Special Care Unit
10. Unplanned returns to the Operating Room

— Maryland Hospital Association (1989). *Executive Summary: MHA Quality Indicator Project, 2 May 1989.* Lutherville, MD: MHA.

When the U.S. federal Health Care Financing Agency (HCFA) published hospital mortality data, it seemed to be proposing that a facility's mortality rate could be used as that "universal quality meter". The validity and comparability of mortality data have been reviled and discussed and universally rejected since that day, but the search for quality meters (in the plural) has continued unabated. Inspecting agencies, third-party payors and hospital boards need yardsticks to measure and compare institutional performance. In their recent book, *The Board's Role in Quality Care,* Orlikoff and Totten list fifty-five "possible indicators of quality for the board" in eight internal and six external categories.[13] More to the point are the lists of ten indicators developed by the Maryland Hospital Association and tested by fourteen multi-hospital systems (Exhibit 3.13) and the twenty indicators that constitute the set used by CCHFA's Outcomes

Exhibit 3.14
CCHFA Outcomes Measurement Project

List of Outcomes

1. **Preadmission Activity** (elective surgery)
   - (a) time interval from admission to OR
   - (b) number and scope of admission delays

2. **Intermediate Outcomes**
   - (a) Special Care Unit — use/type/duration
   - (b) DNR order present
   - (c) Adverse in-patient occurrences (21 types/date)
   - (d) Adverse intraoperative occurrences (21 types/date)
   - (e) Return to OR
   - (f) Trauma suffered in hospital
   - (g) Nosocomial infection
   - (h) Prolonged stay

3. **Discharge Planning**
   - (a) Urinary and bowel elimination at discharge
   - (b) Mobility at discharge
   - (c) Alimentation at discharge
   - (d) Discharge therapies, including IV therapy, oxygen, dialysis, implants, monitoring, medications, dressings, orthopaedic and physiotherapy
   - (e) Care giver
   - (f) Follow-up plan
   - (g) Discharge disposition

4. **Final Outcomes**
   - (a) Death
   - (b) Readmission
   - (c) Long LOS

— Canadian Council on Health Facilities Accreditation (October 1989). *Quality Assurance: The Future (Outcomes Measurement Project).* Ottawa: CCHFA.

Measurement Project in Canada (Exhibit 3.14). The third list of global indicators shown comes from three community hospitals near Toronto that have been sharing comparable data on fourteen indicators quarterly for more than five years (Exhibit 3.15), while many other more prestigious agencies and groups have created and abandoned similar lists or sets of indicators. Although indicator sets will come and go — and the interest of both accreditation bodies, CCHFA and JCAHO, will probably wane as continuous quality improvement becomes more of a reality — the thirst for Wyszewianski's quality meters will continue. In an indicator society, people search for indicators descriptive of everything they value.

Exhibit 3.15
Tri-Hospital Quality Indicators

Surgical in-patient cancellation rate

Long-term care occupancy

In-patient autopsy rate

Employee sick time rate

Adult death rate

Newborn death rate

Caesarean section rate

Stillbirth rate

Employee incident severity rate

Surgical wound infection rate

Postoperative death rate < 48 h

Hospital complication rate

No. of medication incidents

Patient incident rate

— Stacey, S., Henderson, M. and Markel, F. (1985). Patient care indicators: Involving trustees in QA. *Hospital Trustee 9* (5 [Sept.-Oct.]):24-26. Also: Thomas, J. (1990). A hospital-wide QA indicator report. *Dimensions 67* (1 [Feb.]):24-27.

3.8
Conclusion

Indicators are not just a further sophistication of an already too-complex QA program. They are used widely for four good reasons. First, their use provides a highly efficient means of monitoring performance; they save time. Second, good indicators are widely comparable — to last month, to other facilities or departments, to industry norms. Third, they can or should be the source of other or further investigations. Fourth, QA indicators integrate well with those of risk management (risk indicators) and utilization review, two strategies integral to health care quality. Indicators are also constructs of the future: indicator use is essential to effective CQI. In his foreword to the Joint Commission's *Primer*, O'Leary writes:

> *Inherent to the ability to continually improve is the need to measure and monitor performance.*[14]

References

1. Canadian Hospital Association *et al.* (1989). *Joint Statement on Outcome-Oriented Indicators of Quality in Health Care Facilities: Recommendations for Action.* Ottawa: CHA, pp. 1 and 6.
2. "Indicator-Driven Monitoring Systems." Custom Education Program for Kingston General Hospital, Kingston, Ontario, 20 September 1990.
3. Joint Commission on Accreditation of Healthcare Organizations (1990). *Primer on Indicator Development and Application: Measuring Quality in Health Care.* Oakbrook Terrace, IL: JCAHO, p. 21.
4. Attributed to J. Elinson.
5. CHA *et al., op. cit.*(see Note 1), p. 4.

6. Steiber, S.R. and Krowinski, W.J. (1990). *Measuring and Managing Patient Satisfaction.* Chicago: American Hospital Association. Also: Cunningham, L. (1991). *The Quality Connection in Health Care: Integrating Patient Satisfaction and Risk Management.* San Francisco: Jossey-Bass.

7. Canadian Council on Health Facilities Accreditation (1992). *Acute Care: Small Community Hospitals.* Ottawa: CCFA.

8. JCAHO, *op. cit.* (see Note 3).

9. Black, M., Van Berkel, C., Green, E., Everett, I. and Krilyk, J. (1989). Criteria map: Potential for skin breakdown. A quality assurance tool for use in any setting. *Quality Review Bulletin (QRB) 15*(11 [Nov.]):340-346.

10. *Collins Dictionary of the English Language* (1986), ed. P. Hanks. Second ed. London: Collins.

11. Cyr, L.V. (1991). Managing for change: A departmental Quality Improvement Program (QIP). *Healthcare Management Forum 4* (3 [Fall]):3-10.

12. Wyszewianski, L. (1988). The emphasis on measurement in quality assurance: Reasons and implications. *Inquiry 25* (Winter):424-436. (Passage cited appears on p. 426.)

13. Orlikoff, J.E. and Totten, M.K. (1991). *The Board's Role in Quality Care: A Practical Guide for Hospital Trustees.* Chicago: American Hospital Association, pp. 103-104.

14. JCAHO, *op. cit.* (see Note 3).

4

The Evaluation of Professional Performance

It is time now to redeem the promise made in Chapter 2 and prescribe the ways in which performance evaluation in quality assurance can best be done. This chapter begins with the proposition that mature QA programs use all of four data sources in assessing quality, then describes each in detail. The chapter concludes with a presentation of the QA Calendar, a scheduling device that allows department heads to anticipate and manage the QA activities of their staff.

One of the messages that I have tried to convey this past year to QA institutes across Ontario is that there are not one but four different sources of data on quality available to most QA programs. This message has been liberating. For many, audit has been their only method of assessment; repeated use has dwarfed these audits, and the pressure of deadlines has narrowed their focus. And what are the topics of these routine and repetitive exercises? Not the outcome or even the process of care, but the incidentals of the process — charting, safety checks, correct procedures. Many department heads and head nurses have become sick to death of repetitive audits and are grateful of the opportunity to use other methods of assessment, provided they are not too time-consuming or complicated. They also like the prospect of asking and answering questions about the outcome of care. People want to know that they are making a difference.

These audiences have learned the new password: PAIX, peace. "In quality assurance what gives me peace of mind is quality data from *patients* or clients, *audits, indicators,* and outside *experts.*" The memory aid PAIX is useful because department heads need to have the four evaluation options in mind when they plan the assessment of a topic or problem. The four sources differ from one another and introduce different types of data and differing viewpoints on professional performance. Audits and indicators are most sympathetic to the professional, inspecting agencies are most authoritative, and patients and clients the least predictable. But all deserve to be heard.

4.1
Audit

People call any study they do in QA an audit and, according to the dictionary, they are correct. Audit is a generic term meaning "any thoroughgoing check or examination".[1] However, in this text I shall use the term in a narrow sense to denote one of three structured activities: the criterion-referenced audit, the focussed study or investigative audit, and (in Chapter 6) the data-based audit.

The Criterion-Referenced Audit

Definition
Although not usually accorded its full title, the criterion-referenced audit is the most common form of audit used in quality assurance. In this audit the department begins with

its criteria or standards; it compares the data on its actual performance with the standards set; it examines the revealed discrepancies before summarizing its results in a report and acting to correct or improve performance. The purpose of a criterion-referenced audit is to validate current or recent past practice. Its findings are expressed in terms of percentage compliance with the standards. The standards themselves can be very broad (e.g., there shall be a written history and physical on the chart within twenty-four hours of admission; any attempt at a history and physical will suffice) or tightly defined (e.g., the result will be correct within one standard deviation of the mean). This spread between broad standards and defined criteria makes the criterion-referenced audit very adaptable. It is particularly useful in examining aspects of *structure* or inputs in the patient care equation (e.g., staff credentials, adequacy of equipment, environmental safety) and *process* or the procedures employed in care (e.g., preparation of the patient for surgery, the step-by-step procedure for changing a sterile dressing or doing a PA chest in Radiology). Criterion-referenced audits are much less successful in examining patient outcome or service outcome. But patient outcome is difficult to assess by any means.

There is a down side to criterion-referenced auditing. First, it can become self-justifying. These audits belong to the professionals who set the standards and perform the processes. Audit and performance can occur in a loop that excludes other people or realities: "The operation was a success, and the patient died." Second, the value of these audits diminishes in direct proportion to the frequency of their repetition. A major value in audits of all kinds lies not in their findings but in their creation. The development of a new audit demands the analysis of practice, an exploration of the literature, and the selection of meaningful and measurable criteria. Experts believe that these preparatory steps result in much more behaviour change than the attribution of audit results to the team or individual clinicians. The third drawback of criterion-referenced auditing is that the need to find measurable aspects of performance tends to narrow the focus of inquiry to the easily measurable, which often means the unimportant. It is always worth reminding quality assurance audiences of the practical truth that the importance of aspects of life is inversely related to the ease of measuring them. The more fundamental and important the issue, the more difficult it is to assess with any degree of precision.

Conduct

Audits are conducted in a series of interlocking steps and, recognizing that in practice sometimes the steps become transposed, we shall describe the conduct of the audit chronologically.

Step 1: Choice of audit team

What is important about the team is that it should be a team; auditing is not an individual activity. Individuals can be accused of making personal judgements about peers, rather than objective judgements on performance. As often, individuals may lack the fortitude to make the judgements that the evidence dictates, because they would prefer to avoid the unpopularity that might ensue. Audit findings must be those of a group, and the group, to be credible, must be drawn from all the same levels and specialities of staff whose performance is under review.

Sometimes team members are chosen because it is "their turn". At other times the department's choice of topic dictates which practitioners should participate because of their expertise. Again there is need for caution. If the audit team consists entirely of experts, those whose performance is being reviewed can question the team's credibility or the application of the standards as being too exacting for non-specialists.

Step 2: Choice of topic

People who complain about the difficulty of finding good audit topics should be heard. I believe it is the hardest task in the audit process; "any old topic" will not do. A good audit topic has the following characteristics:

- It is *significant.* If an audit team is to spend expensive time on a topic, that topic must be a significant aspect of performance. To convey a sense of priority, the CCHFA uses the terms outcome-related, high-value, high-risk and problem-prone.

- It is *relevant,* first to the investigators and the team from which they are drawn. The topic must, even in its planning stage, offer the team important insights, support or confirmation. I sometimes ask audit planners to write a "buy-in statement" — a compelling reason to choose the topic, gather the data and carry the audit to completion. The validation of ho-hum clinical routines can be counted on to frustrate busy, motivated people.

- The topic in its final form must be *measurable,* by which two things are meant: there are data available (or retrievable), and the topic is so focussed that the project can be completed within a limited time frame. My recommended period from team formation to audit report is ninety days.

Step 3: Choice of method
An audit team will not know what method of investigation it will need until the topic is chosen and all the possible sources of data have been identified. The best data are those already available. The next best are those that can be collected without too much trouble, and the least favourable data are those that have to be mined specially. Most audit teams will be faced with two alternatives: the criterion-referenced audit (to validate current and technical performance) and the focussed study or investigative audit (to analyze and improve present performance). Does the team want to know How good?, or ask the questions What? and Why? (We will examine the sequence of a focussed study in the next section of this chapter.)

Step 4: Development (and adoption) of a criteria set
One of the worst things that can happen to an audit team is

the rejection of its audit criteria when it presents its report. This can happen if the audit team fails to insist on adequate discussion, and adoption, of the performance criteria that provide the foundations of the judgements to be made. Audit criteria need to be adopted formally at a staff meeting by a show of hands and recorded in the minutes.

Step 5: Data retrieval and analysis

There are four functions connected with the audit data or evidence of performance. Retrospective data can be *retrieved* — charts pulled, diaries and logs found, and rejects or repeats segregated. This is a mechanical function and need not be done by the professional unless the rules of confidentiality require it. Second is the task of *analysis,* in which a sort is made between those items that meet one specification or another. Again, this too can be quite routine, as the health record analyst identifies the cases meeting the criteria set, and those that are outliers. Similarly, a pharmacy technician can identify drug labels that meet specifications and those that do not. These tasks are ideal for a leader to share with members of the audit committee.

Step 6: Evaluation and reporting

Data evaluation and reporting are professional and managerial responsibilities. It is the peers, i.e., the professionals whose performance is under scrutiny, who should make the professional judgement on the evidence. They should look at the outliers to estimate the clinical appropriateness of deviating from the standards chosen. Similarly, the professionals need to make their own judgements on the significance of the evidence. These judgements can range from satisfaction to severe dissatisfaction. The team's evaluation will fuel its action plan; if its judgements are mild, its actions will be conservative.

The duty to report is a function of management. Staff can undertake all other audit functions. Reports should be honest and incisive, and identify systems that worked or did not work, but not health care workers nor their patients. Confidentiality respects human dignity; cover-up offends all.

Step 7: Quality improvement

In the old days QA said, "... and *if necessary,* remedy, reaudit and report." Today the injunction is, "Even within the good performance, identify opportunities for improving the processes of care or service." Such opportunities should be recognized by the audit team, discussed with the department, and the improvements introduced as soon as convenient, one step at a time.

There are more complete and authoritative descriptions of the audit process.[2] The description above reveals my own biases: the insistence on topic significance and practitioner buy-in, the choice of small samples, short timetables, and full participation. Good audits are interesting and rewarding.

The Focussed Study

During a QA workshop I recently led, a group of professional departments in a teaching hospital proposed the following audit topics for consideration:

1. An audit to identify level of patient satisfaction with splints made for carpal tunnel syndrome (Occupational Therapy).

2. An audit to evaluate the effectiveness of an Out-patient Pain Management Program in terms of improvement in function (Physiotherapy).

3. An audit of Discharge Planning time from receipt of referral to sending out required forms and the identification of factors affecting length of time taken (Social Work).

4. An audit of the quality of workmanship in the fabrication of a device for patients to wear in the ear during swimming (Audiology).

5. An audit of the extent to which patient care goals are met after a specific number of weeks of therapy (Psychology).

Social Work's topic could easily be evaluated by means of a criterion-referenced audit. Criteria would probably include elapsed time and items detailing the appropriate documentation. Following audit, the department could list common causes of delay through an examination of outliers.

Before Audiology can use a criterion-referenced audit to assess quality of workmanship, it will need to develop measurable criteria to describe it. Evaluation will more likely be based on expert opinion or peer assessment of the hearing device, as well as patient satisfaction.

Occupational Therapy (patient satisfaction), Physiotherapy (effectiveness of treatment) and Psychology (goal attainment in therapy) will all seek a more flexible method of inquiry or assessment: the focussed study or investigative audit.

The focussed study is an inductive method of assessment in which the department begins with the data and draws from them conclusions about quality. Quality may include effectiveness, fitness for use, appropriateness to the patient, accuracy, satisfaction and many other judgements besides. The special feature of the focussed study is its flexibility. In QA our bias is towards outcome, in spite of the difficulty of measuring or assessing it. We will come closer to assessing the outcome (or features of it) using the focussed study than any other method. An example may help.

During the workshop for which the list of five audit topics was prepared, OT decided to plan an audit to investigate the carpal tunnel splinting. In doing so they enlarged the focus of their audit beyond simple patient satisfaction. They decided to:

- go to the charts
    to identify the patients in the study
    to assess the clinical necessity of the splinting
    to document the duration of the splinting;

- inspect the splinting on the patient
    to check its level of support
    to make other (peer) professional judgements about
        form and positioning;

- ask the patient about comfort (absence of pain), ability to use the hand, level of convenience and other matters.

With this variety of questions and its interest in examining the fitted splint, the department could be satisfied with a small sample and a short time frame.

In a focussed study the department is interested in knowing what is happening or has happened, and why. It can go to as many data sources as are readily available. In drawing its conclusions, the department will take the extra step in order to answer the question: What can we do to improve our care/service/product?

The steps to be followed in both the criterion-referenced audit and the focussed study are detailed in a group of exhibits. Exhibit 4.1 lists the opening steps in developing an audit, leading to the choice of audit method. Exhibit 4.2 describes the steps taken in the conduct of a criterion-referenced audit, and Exhibit 4.3 those necessary to a focussed study. The concluding steps common to both, or all — when a data-based review is included — are listed in Exhibit 4.4.

4.2
Using Indicators in Performance Assessment

After devoting an entire chapter to the development of indicators, we need only to integrate their use with the other three methods of performance assessment. Department managers will:

1. Investigate and address each sentinel event as it occurs.

2. Record, on a run chart each period, the total number of sentinel events or category of events.

Exhibit 4.1
Planning Protocol for Audit

---

1. **Choice of Topic**
   Which of the following criteria does the topic meet:
   - ❏ Patient-centred
   - ❏ High-risk
   - ❏ High-volume
   - ❏ Problem-prone
   - ❏ Interservice

2. **Choice of Audit Team**
   Names:
   Are all levels of staff involved in the performance under review represented on the team?

3. **Setting Objectives**
   The objects of the audit are:
   - •
   - •
   - •

4. **Leading Questions**
   List the questions that need to be answered:
   - •
   - •
   - •

5. **Choice of Audit Method**
   Select ONE:
   - ❏ Criterion-referenced audit (to validate quality of present performance)
   - ❏ Focussed study (to investigate a problem/performance area)
   - ❏ Data-based review (comparative study utilizing HMRI or other electronic data base)

6. **Validation**
   Is the team sure that the benefits of carrying out the proposed study outweigh the costs of undertaking it? If not: reconsider/refocus topic to one that promises direct benefit to practitioners.

Exhibit 4.2
The Criterion-Referenced Audit

#1-6   See Planning Protocol for Audit (Exhibit 4.1)

7.   **Development of Criteria List**

Activity/Practice under Review	Criteria of Performance	Authority

1.

2.

   (Use separate sheet.)

n

8.   **Available Data**

In the order of the criteria list (#7), list the data available and their source.

Criteria	Data Source

1.

2.

   (Use separate sheet.)

n

Delete from criteria list those which cannot be reviewed with the data available.

9.   **Audit Sample**

Cases:

Period:

Sample should be identified by numbers of cases and period(s) from which they are drawn. If total sample is not intended, how will cases be selected from total?

10.   **Criteria Acceptance**

Give plans to share audit criteria with staff whose practice will be subject to review. Are the criteria acceptable to them? If not: review, explain, revise.

(Proceed to Audit Management #11-15 [Exhibit 4.4])

Exhibit 4.3

The Focussed Study (Investigative Audit)

#1-6   See Planning Protocol for Audit

7. **Problem Statement**

    A one-paragraph statement of the focus of the audit (problem/topic):

8. **Available Data**

    Indicate data source(s) available for review. (Remember: patients/clients, indicators, external agencies.)

    Data   Source

9. **Diagnostic Journey**

    There are several methods of analyzing problems:

    ❏   Process Flow Chart   ❏   Brainstorming
    ❏   Cause-and-Effect Diagram   ❏   Scatter Plots

    There are several methods of displaying data:

    ❏   Run Charts   ❏   Pie Charts
    ❏   Histograms/Bar Charts   ❏   Pareto Charts

    Indicate which (or other) method(s) you will use.

10. **List other departments that should be consulted or could have information to contribute.**

    (Proceed to Audit Management #11-15 [Exhibit 4.4])

---

3. Record, on run charts each period, the department's rate of occurrence of its various rate-based indicators, and review their significance.

4. Report the department's performance according to its indicators to the superior each period. The frequency of

Exhibit 4.4
Audit Management

---

11. **Indicate who will carry out the data abstractions and timetable proposed:**

    Abstractors:

    Proposed completion date:

12. **Analysis of data**

    Consideration of outliers: Peers -

    Proposed completion date:

13. **Evaluation**

    Proposal for remedial action/quality improvement steps:

    -
    -
    -
    -

14. **Preparation of report**

    Circulation date:

    Presentation date:

15. **Date of reaudit or proposal of further/follow-up study.**

---

reporting indicators is primarily determined by the volume of data. The general rule is that indicators are reviewed and reported monthly. Some departments or some indicators will simply not generate enough data for meaningful review on a monthly basis. The rule for them will be quarterly reporting.

5. Annually revisit each indicator, by means of a focussed study, to investigate the performance underlying the rate or number of events. The intent is to stagger these revisits over the year and do them singly or, if the indicators are related, in groups.

This sequence of record, review, report and revisit points again to the usefulness and efficiency of indicators. This data source has three uses: concurrent monitoring, information flow, and problem finding.

4.3
Integrating Expert Opinion in Quality Assessment

Hospitals are rightly among the most inspected and reviewed agencies in our society. The personal and physical vulnerability of the patient, the need for individuation in care, and the power and discretion modern medicine has placed in the hands of care givers all provide justification for society's concern about what goes on in hospitals.

Hospitals are reviewed and inspected according to their multiple personalities: they are at once hotels, employers, health clinics, schools and businesses. Exhibit 4.5 gives a partial listing of inspecting agencies. These contribute to the hospital's assessment of how well it performs its various roles by their sheer number and variety, as well as by their reports enhancing or challenging the assurance of quality. The only problem is how to integrate outside agency reports into the hospital's QA program. I recommend three steps.

Notification

Although the hospital in its many aspects is inspected (or its data reviewed) frequently, notice of such inspections or their reports is often not given to senior management, or given by senior management to the board. This silence indicates not a cover-up by the departments inspected, but rather a lack of

Exhibit 4.5
Hospital Inspection Agencies

Hospital as Clinic
Hospital Medical Records Institute (HMRI)
Laboratory Proficiency Testing Program (LPTP) — OMA
Radiation Protection Branch — Ministry of Health (MOH)
Laboratory Licencing Branch — MOH
Coroner's Office

Hospital as Employer
Ministry of Labour
Workers Compensation Board
Human Rights Commission

Hospital as School
Colleges, universities, and professional colleges
accrediting/teaching internship and residency programs

Hospital as Hotel
Public Health Department
Fire Marshall
Grand Jury
Insurance companies (boiler inspection)

Hospital as Business
Financial auditors
Public Trustee
Blue Cross

All Aspects
Canadian Council on Health Facilities Accreditation
Ministry of Health

awareness that others might be interested in what to them is routine. For example, it is easier for a large laboratory to know which months (if any) it will *not* test quality control for the Laboratory Proficiency Testing Program (LPTP) than the months it will test. Similarly, it is unlikely that the Chief Engineer will register with his or her superior when the hospital's boilers are due for annual inspection, or the Director of Food Services to report on the frequency of the visits of the Public Health Inspector. So our first advice to department heads is that these inspections are an essential part of their QA programs, and that management needs to be apprised of their scheduling (or, if random, of their occurrence). Regular inspections can be registered on the QA Calendar described later in this chapter.

Translation

After more than twenty-five years working in and around hospitals, I have never seen a QA report incorporating data from LPTP. I have seen LPTP reports and scatter plots, but never an explanation of results in lay terms.

If staff intend to share data that have long been of professional interest only, such information must come with its own legend.

Report

It is proposed that departments subject to outside review should report all inspections, whether or not senior management or the board express interest in them. Irregular or unscheduled inspections should be reported when they occur; others can be summarized in the department's regular quarterly report. Needless to say, such reports will carry details of the ways in which discovered discrepancies have been addressed.

4.4
Hearing from
Patients

One of the central weaknesses in Canadian quality assurance is the silence of the client or customer of health care: the patient. Probably only a small minority of departmental programs incorporate patient data in the assessment of health services, and perhaps seventy-five per cent of such data is drawn from precoded self-completion questionnaires. In this section we need to address the value or usefulness of approaching patients for their views, to look at the variety of ways of eliciting patient data, and to describe what patient responses can contribute to quality of service. In postscript, we should provide advice to departments who serve professional or non-patient clients.

The Value of Listening to Patients

A particular strength in British quality assurance has been its insistence on hearing first from the client. This demand has been sounded by the Chief Executive in Whitehall and picked up in regions and districts throughout the National Health Service. The white paper *Working for Patients* [3] and the Personal Service Initiative of the Trent Region are examples of this focus. In contrast, Canadian QA has tended to be supercilious about the value of patient perceptions. We have wanted patients to be happy but have been uncertain of the accuracy or usefulness of their views. Now we are on notice that we must listen to our patients or clients. As we shall see, continuous quality improvement (CQI) insists that the client is king. According to CQI we are first to listen to our clients; second, to meet their expressed needs; and third, to meet the needs we might have if we, the experts, were the patient.

In 1989 Goldfield and Nash edited a collection of papers for the American College of Physicians, entitled *Providing Quality Care: The Challenge to Physicians*. In summarizing a paper by Kaplan and Ware, "The Patient's Role in Health Care and Quality Assessment," the editors wrote:

> *Kaplan and Ware challenge one of the basic tenets of modern medicine — care is too technical and scientifically based to be evaluated by patients. They show, rather convincingly, that the evidence favours patients' abilities to judge not only the interpersonal skills of physicians (what used to be called bedside manner) but their technical prowess as well. Consumers of health care services have become more discerning shoppers; patients are demanding a more active decision-making role in their care. Clinicians ought to pay attention to these demands and to the skills patients demonstrate by evaluating what physicians do.*[4]

Not only are patients competent in their judgements about care givers; Kaplan and Ware point out that the more patients are able to participate in their own care, the better they fare. They cite studies in support of the propositions that (1) informed patients do better than those who are less informed about their condition and plan of care and (2) those patients who are given an opportunity to participate in the choice of therapy do better than those who are expected simply to consent. In this context, listening to patients is first and foremost good patient care and only secondarily an activity useful to quality assurance. Or, to put it another way: Listening to patients is a necessity of care; using insights from patients in quality assurance is both an option and perhaps a skill that needs to be acquired.

In the United States this obligation of staff to heed their patients' needs for information and autonomy is enshrined in a new accreditation chapter on patient rights.[5] In a British monograph, McIver[6] points out that service evaluation and patient education are just two of nine important purposes in seeking the views of patients. She lists, in addition:

- *Planning service provision.* The fullest discussion that can occur between potential client and service provider will offer the best chance of achieving an appropriate service.

- *Setting service standards.* Gaining consumer input into the professional definition of standards to be achieved.

- *Monitoring service standards.* The validation of service quality through the regular reception of feedback from clients.

- *Service review.* Assessing the viability of the service following major changes in its delivery or context.

- *Public relations.* Enhancing the views of the public about a service through demonstrating openness.

- *Customer relations.* Improving the relationship that exists between clients and service providers.

- *Purchaser and provider relations.* Mapping the relations between different NHS health entities in the light of operating contracts in the 1990s.

Methods to Obtain Patients' Views

McIver adopts a useful distinction between methods that yield quantitative versus qualitative data. She describes quantitative methods as

> *[those involving] the collection and analysis of information in numerical form. That is, incidence or rates of occurrences — death rates, accident rates, throughput figures, the number of patients answering 'yes' to a particular question, etc.*[7]

She reviews three methods of quantitative data gathering: the precoded self-completion questionnaire, the population survey ("of people who are not current users of health services") and the structured interview. Perhaps only the first is relevant to QA as opposed to health services research. Many hospitals give patients, or mail to ex-patients, generic questionnaires. Hospital associations and groups sometimes develop such questionnaires. These and others developed by individual hospitals are often reviewed in the literature.[8]

Questionnaires and interviews reappear on McIver's list of qualitative methods, which she describes as those involving "the collection and analysis of narrative information." In this context, however, both would rely upon open-ended questions and the service provider's analysis or interpretation of the varied responses received. Including questionnaires and interviews, McIver lists eleven methods of obtaining qualitative data.

When I put the question of how to obtain patient data to a QA conference at the King's Fund Centre in London, participants listed fifteen ways of getting feedback from patients or families (see Exhibit 4.6). Their extensive list contrasts markedly with Canadian QA's overdependence on patient satisfaction surveys (#2) and complaints and commendations (#4). Many of these will occur in the four-category description that follows.

Patients' opinions can be obtained by watching them (observation), recognizing patient views expressed in formal settings (recognition), asking their help (direct methods), and listening to those who would speak for them (advocacy).

Observation

Much can be learned from watching people cope with their environment or the particular demands of their situation. Prior to remodelling its out-patient department, one hospital had a staff member sit in the clinic and watch who came and went, how long they stayed, how they coped with registration and appointment booking, what they did about meals, what part was played by relatives and how they got home. Observation is perhaps used more widely in QA than we remember: noting patient participation rates, "no

Exhibit 4.6
Methods of Collecting Feedback from Patients/Clients

1. Patients' council (in Canada, residents' council)

2. Satisfaction survey

3. Direct communication (staff listening and asking questions)

4. Complaints and commendations

5. Family conferences

6. Weekend-pass questionnaire (debriefing psychiatric patients on their return to hospital following a weekend out)

7. Journal entries (notations about the behaviour of Alzheimer patients attending a day hospital program)

8. *Brown's Beat* — a patient-run newspaper

9. Patient rounds

10. Phone calls to patients (made by the facility's chief executive)

11. Postoperative day-surgery questionnaire

12. Observation

13. Volunteer follow-up phone call/interview

14. Care giver questionnaire

15. Unit procedure manual

— As suggested by British QA professionals, 25 June 1991. Explanations in parentheses have been added by C.R.M. Wilson.

shows", tray returns (food not consumed), and new mothers bathing their babies would all be commonly used forms of client observation. Staff are always observing their patients and responding to them. All too often these observations do not become data usable in QA, because once the situation is observed and, if necessary, remedied, the data are lost. For this reason, departments and nursing units are advised to keep a patient/case journal in which staff are encouraged to note patients' problems of care or coping and record patient/client questions when they arise.

Recognition

There are four entries on the feedback list in Exhibit 4.6 that involve staff taking note of patient activity: the patients'/ residents' council, a patient-run newspaper, conferences with families and clinical rounds. To these should be added the insights that come from therapeutic and support groups organized for patients (AIDS, transplant, coronary rehabilitation, spinal cord injury, rape victims, terminal cancer patients) and families (care givers, the bereaved, addict families, trauma families). Staff who are interested in improving, rather than simply measuring, quality will recognize that activities such as these can provide authentic information. As with observation, the trick is not in seeing but retaining the incident or response so as to analyze it and related data, and address them.

Direct Methods

Interview

It is easy to let the negatives obscure the usefulness of staff questioning patients. Interviews are expensive in terms of time and, depending on their anxiety level, patients may tell staff what they think staff want to hear. On the other hand, a good interview may be worth ten or twenty questionnaires, and their timing can be arranged to coincide with periods of low patient anxiety. Interviews can be carried out by trained volunteers who are not authority figures, and be done over the phone when patients are in the security of their own homes.

Many large retailers in the United States have given up formal market research in favour of daily interaction with their clients.[9] We could take a leaf from their book. Instead of conducting a few multitopic interviews a department could, for a limited period, ask all its clients the same open-ended question, and record their answers verbatim ("What single thing will you remember about your visit to X-ray this morning?" or "Would you suggest one way in which we could have looked after you better today?").

Petersen[10] recommends the use of the following questions in daily interactions to monitor patient satisfaction:

1. What do you expect from your care giver today?

2. How satisfied were you with your care today?

The use of interview is particularly relevant when staff want to gauge the outcome of treatment. Patients can talk about the presence or absence of pain, use and degree of comfort/discomfort with prostheses (splints and casts, hearing aids, seats, shoes and implants, e.g., hips and knees). To the extent that patients were involved in goal setting, they can also be questioned as to their progress and future goals.

Whatever the question(s) asked, staff need to do two things: respond to the patient's answer appropriately so as to improve care then and there, and second, record and forward the patient's response for later collation and analysis with data from the whole sample.

Questionnaire

Interviews are but one of several direct methods of gaining data on patient experience. In-patients can, shortly before discharge, be given short self-completion questionnaires that contain enough open-ended questions to allow them to give the messages they want to give.

Exhibit 4.6 mentions four different client groups as being polled by questionnaires: in-patients (#2), weekend release (#6), day surgery (#11) and family care giver (#14). Questionnaire design is a sophisticated skill. For example, some survey experts insist that "designing surveys without first asking customers which survey variables matter most to them elicits management-driven — not customer-driven — data."[11] For this reason, as well as the need to protect patients from annoyance, it is recommended that all questionnaires be reviewed for form and content and authorized by the facility's QA committee, which should also agree with the choice of sample to be polled.

Focus Groups

Patients and families can be invited to participate in focus group discussion of their experience of the hospital and the services provided for them. These discussions are an opportunity for staff to learn about what they and others have and have not done, and to gain insights as to how the hospital system(s) can be changed, the better to meet the needs of clients. There is a narrow line between focus groups and therapeutic and support groups; the distinction is one of intent. The intent of a focus group is to look at the adequacy, appropriateness and sensitivity of the system to the needs of the client.

Patient Logs/Diaries

Finally, patients and families can be encouraged to keep notes about their experience, so that they can track their illness and its seasons and their sense of comfort or discomfort with the system of care and its provision. These logs or diaries will be useful to staff when they want to look at the effects of patient education and the compliance of out-patients with dietary, medication and exercise prescriptions. Newly diagnosed maturity-onset diabetics, new mothers, sports injury patients and postoperative coronary bypass patients would be good candidates for diary keeping.

The intent of this discussion is to invite QA leaders to want to hear from their patients/clients and to be creative in gathering data from them. Three notes conclude this section. First, authorities in this area have discovered a strong correlation between patient satisfaction and (their) perception of quality.[12] Second, patient satisfaction is strongly conditioned by patient expectation; thus, time spent on creating realistic expectations is important. Third is the oft-repeated reminder that all departments have clients who can be observed, listened to, questioned and surveyed, although all do not have patients or external clients.

Advocacy

In most health care systems there are advocates or representatives of all patients or groups of patients. These people or associations, with or without the patients' consent, represent them and the needs they believe patients to have. Whether health care professionals like it or not, they live in the age of advocacy, victims and empowerment. The essential fact in quality assurance is that these representatives may contribute valuable information about patients, their experience and their care. It is worth listing some examples:

- *Ombudsmen/patient representatives.* Some hospitals fund such a position on their staff. In others, patient and family complaints are handled for the Chief Executive by Public Relations or — sensibly, in some cases — by the Risk Management office.

- *Patient advocate.* This is the title of a post obligatory in all provincial psychiatric hospitals in Ontario. The advocate, who reports directly to the hospital's Community Advisory Board, looks into all patient complaints and protects the civil rights of psychiatric in-patients.

- *Hospital chaplains and social workers* often describe part of their authorized function as patient advocacy, both with other hospital staff and in gaining access to community services and support.

In addition, there are many voluntary associations dedicated to the amelioration of the often tragic situations of physically, emotionally and cognitively challenged individuals. Although physicians, nurses and trustees all see themselves in the role of patient advocate, credibility today often goes to the outsider. This can be galling, but hospital people have to develop the ability to perceive truths about quality and appropriateness in spite of the noise and rancour that often accompany them.

The Contribution of Patient Experience to Quality of Care

We can make five statements about the value of patient evaluation of care within the context of the quality assurance program.

1. Patient data are readily available and not difficult or time-consuming to gather and use. If staff ask, patients will tell them.

2. Patient evaluations are judgements from an authentic and independent source and will corroborate or challenge the staff-developed evaluations reached by audit, indicator review or even an outside agency.

3. Patient comments often do not fit the departmental concerns which are the focus of most of QA. Instead, patients focus on systems failures or breakdowns. Cunningham has isolated six major areas of patient dissatisfaction: professional inattentiveness, delays in care, unrealistic expectations, poor communication among staff and with patient, unprofessional behaviour in staff, and breakdown in the continuity of care.[13] None of these is department- or profession-specific.

4. Dialogue with patients concerning their condition and the appropriateness of the care they are receiving is, if Kaplan and Ware are to be believed, first and foremost good patient care. Such dialogue is a ready form of concurrent monitoring, and its insights make possible and imperative immediate correction or amelioration.

5. Finally, lay trustees find patient data very convincing —
   as they should. When all the professional language stops
   and the organizational cloud bank lifts, what do the
   patients — the real people from "my" street — say?

These arguments provide justification for the PIER
model's insistence that no departmental QA program
(including Medical) can be considered satisfactory which
does not employ patient or client data in its evaluation of
care at least once per year.

Involving Non-Patient Clients in Service Evaluation

There are, of course, many departments whose primary
clients are not patients but professionals or line departments.
Obvious examples would be Medical Records, many
laboratories, Materiel Management, Human Resources, and
Engineering & Plant Maintenance. Others have more than
one important client, such as Radiology/Diagnostic Imaging
and Pharmacy. Fortunately we have progressed beyond the
days when department status was determined by proximity
to the patient's bed. All departments have vital roles to play.

The other advance in our thinking is more recent and
comes to us from CQI, namely, that all employees play three
roles: as customers of others from whom they receive
information, resources and material; as processors as they act
on what they have received, making their contribution to the
product or service; and as suppliers, as they hand off to
another the product they have worked on. In QA, this means
that supplier departments can and should provide their
customer departments with the opportunity to evaluate or
rate the service they receive.

Supplier departments can adopt several of the strategies
outlined above with reference to patient satisfaction.
Moreover, they should do so at least once a year. Three
simple examples must suffice. Human Resources could

decide to interview (with four to six open-ended questions) six department heads and head nurses, concerning the service management and staff received on personnel matters. The Radiology department of a small hospital which had to send its radiographs to a medical centre for reading asked the consultant radiologists to rate the quality of their films on four or five aspects in comparison with films read from other hospitals. Once or twice a year the manager of Materiel Management might attend a portion of a head nurse or department head meeting to discuss the department's past performance and possible future service. These examples use a questionnaire, a service/product rating, and a focus group opportunity.

4.5
Pulling It All Together: The QA Calendar

This is the conclusion of both this chapter and this book's first section devoted to the PIER model. It includes some repetition of key concepts and the presentation of a simple instrument through which quality assurance programs are managed.

To begin with first principles, quality assurance is an information system that allows a department or hospital to answer regularly the questions, How well are we doing our job? and How do we know? The job is defined in QA in terms of principal functions (and their important components), all of which are client-focussed. The knowing depends on the continuous evaluation of performance with reference to patients/clients, audits, indicators, and external agencies. QA is expected to be a continuous program of assessment and one that is comprehensive in scope. No department can make an authoritative statement about its performance on the basis of one audit, inspection or survey. Instead, it is intended that over the course of a year the performance of all the principal functions will be assessed by the various means described in this chapter.

The problem we have arrived at is how to organize audits and functions, indicators and interviews in such a way that they yield conclusions about performance and, along the way, provide insights important to practitioners. An information system about care can never be half so important as the care itself. Thus QA needs to be efficient in its use of practitioner time and, through the information it produces, a value-adding system and not simply a tax on time.

Development

The QA Calendar presented in this section was developed by the author for the medical staff of a small hospital in northwestern Ontario. In a succession of meetings with the Chief of Staff and chair of the Tissue & Audit committee, several ongoing medical staff activities had been isolated and labelled as components of an organized QA program. For example, the staff were doing regular chart reviews and criterion audits, and holding educational (CME) sessions with visiting specialists. The Tissue & Audit committee reviewed operative tissue, complications and consents, and supervised death reviews. The staff had also identified its principal functions, which included the clinical supervision of satellite stations. But where was the vehicle? It all looked like so many automobile parts laid out on the garage floor. However, three things were obvious to me: we needed to exploit to the fullest whatever QA-related activities the medical staff were engaged in. Second, the staff needed an ongoing plan rather than haphazard reporting; and third, one activity per month was the upper limit of possible compliance. So the Calendar was born. On it we scheduled the reporting of one committee activity per month and inter-spersed expensive activities (such as audits) with continuous activities (such as chart reviews). In addition, in faithfulness to principal functions, I had to suggest ways in which Nursing Station support could be assessed once a year.

The 1992 version of the QA Calendar is a little more sophisticated than that developed in Sioux Lookout in 1989, but it is still simple in concept. Moreover, if participants in my courses and workshops are to be believed, it is a powerful integrator of the myriad activities that seem to buzz around in quality assurance. When I was writing *Hospital-wide Quality Assurance (HQA),* another author warned me that there would be things I would wish I could revise, but would not be able to, once they were in print. The QA Calendar is presented here as a correction of the one *HQA* strategy I would like to remove from the book. The method of QA planning [14] looks far better in print than it is in practice. Its complexity came home to me when working with a social service agency whose managers balked at the unnecessary intellectual effort it required. I think they would be more pleased with the QA Calendar.

Structure

The QA Calendar (Exhibit 4.7) consists of four columns. The first, obviously, carries the months of the year — the fiscal, academic or calendar year, at the facility's choice. The second column is labelled Management and can carry a range of information relevant to the QA program.

- *Workload.* It is important that departments begin their management of QA by determining when other factors will prevent them from undertaking what I call expensive (i.e., time-consuming) QA activities. Thus it would be appropriate for managers to enter in this column such probable distractions as budget preparation, annual audit (finance), accreditation survey (all), computerization, and times when staffing is problematical, e.g. July/August vacations and the year-end holiday season.

Exhibit 4.7
The Departmental QA Calendar

Month	Management	Audit	Other Reviews: P/I/X
January			
February			
March			
April			
May			
June			
July			
August			
September			
October			
November			
December			

- *Reporting schedule.* It makes obvious sense to mark on the Calendar the months when the department is expected to report its QA activities. Even when a facility adopts a pattern of quarterly reporting, it usually staggers these reports so that the QA committee does not have to review them all at once.

- *Inspections.* Earlier in this chapter I recommended that departments that were subject to regularly scheduled inspections (or submission of data for external review) should enter these occasions on their QA Calendar. These entries belong in the Management column.

The third column is labelled Audits, and should be completed next. The expectation is that all departments will make four entries in this column, i.e., carry out four criterion-referenced audits or focussed studies per annum. There is nothing magical about this number, but four means one per quarter, and three seems a bit light for a continuing activity. But what about five or, better, six — one every two months? If four is good, isn't six much better? My answer is no. The QA Calendar has the functions of both saying how much is expected of a department's program and setting limits — saying when. No one in QA says when "enough is enough". Through the Calendar, the facility can set some limits. Of course, no one is being altruistic in setting limits. We protect the quality of audits by demanding that they be done regularly but infrequently. There is one caveat: audits entered in this column are new inquiries or reaudits after at least a year. Focussed studies of indicator data do not belong here, but in column four.

Three performance assessment activities are entered in the column labelled P/I/X — standing, of course, for patients (clients), indicators, and external agencies. Whenever the department intends to approach its clients for their assessment, wants to review the data underlying an indicator, or expects to report on a scheduled inspection, it will enter a note to that effect in this column.

Content

When possible, each entry in columns 3 and 4 should give the following details: the number of the principal function under review (e.g., #1, #6) and the method of assessment (e.g., CRA = criterion-referenced audit; FS = focussed study); in column 4, P = patient or family, C = client, IR = indicator review, XR = external review. When these columns are completed, their entries should show that the department has scheduled the following:

- The examination of an aspect of all their principal functions, with additional entries for those judged to be more important.

- Four audits in column 3.

- At least one P or C entry denoting the department's intention of approaching its patients or clients for their views or assessment.

- One entry for each month.

Three advisory comments:

First, in small hospitals or small departments (i.e., fewer than five staff) it is unrealistic to expect that staff will be able to maintain a schedule such as that outlined, plus report six to eight indicators per month. Instead, it is better to ask them to monitor and maintain their indicators monthly and do one additional QA activity per quarter, including at least one audit and one patient/client assessment.

Second, management may want to reserve two months for its own purposes. There is merit in the QA committee holding one month when it can ask all departments to carry out an exercise based on a new demand or change in the hospital-wide program. It will also be beneficial for all departments to assess — and report — their readiness for accreditation. They will do this by responding to the current accreditation standards, noting their discrepancies, and proposing an action plan to address them.

Finally, the QA Calendar should be completed in pencil. It is not a final document, though it is filed with management and the QA committee. It belongs to the department and is an aspect of its management of its own program.

Examples of some departmental QA Calendars are included as addenda to this chapter. Exhibit 4.8 was completed by the administrative manager of a Radiology department, although some of the labels are my own. Exhibit 4.9 was completed with me by the nurse manager of a Surgical unit. We walked through the planning process, beginning with the principal functions of her unit, important components, and indicators before putting the ingredients together in the Calendar. The third example (Exhibit 4.10) comes from Human Resources, and was my suggestion for the Personnel department in a medium-sized hospital. None of them should be taken as a prescription. They are practical answers for local situations.

When presenting the QA Calendar I usually refer to two of its particular merits: first, of course, it allows the department to integrate all of its QA activities into an action plan, and thereby questions the necessity of any QA structure that is not directly related to an entry on the Calendar. Second, by forcing the department to anticipate its QA activities, it improves its planning, delegation and use of lead time. The result is usually better-quality audits and other assessments, and less (and more convenient) time devoted to all aspects of the program. But then planners have always told those who would listen that planning saves time and improves performance.

Exhibit 4.8

Quality Assurance Calendar, Department of Radiology

Month	Management	Audit	Other Reviews: P/I/X
January	Budget		Reporting quality and time (I) [#3]
February		Film filing and retrieval audit (CRA) [#4]	
March	Report QA		Review of risk incidents (I) [#2] and waiting time (I) [#2]
April		MD review of film quality (CRA) [#1]	
May			Review of HARP inspection report (X) [#5]
June	Report QA	Procedure audit (positioning, technique, etc.; FS) [#1]	
July	Vacations		Process or QC (I) [#5]
August	Vacations		Spare
September	Report QA		Patient interview/ questionnaire (P) [#2]
October		Audit of procedures for handling infirm patients (FS) [#2]	
November			Review of retakes (I)[#1]
December	Report QA Holidays		Accreditation readiness review

Principal functions:
1. Taking films [April, June, November]
2. Patient handling [March, September, October]
3. Reporting [January]
4. Film library [February]
5. Safety (QC) [May, July]

Exhibit 4.9
Quality Assurance Calendar — Surgical Ward

Month	Management	Audit	Other Reviews: P/I/X
January	Budget		Credentials (I) [#2]
February			Review of surgical delays (I) [#6]
March	R	Nursing dx. [#2]	
April			Review of mo. scores, bedside audit (I) [#3]
May		Effectiveness of pre-op. teaching [#3]	
June	R		Family Qu adequacy of personal care (P) [#3]
July	Vacations		Report on NCPs (I) [#1, #5]
August	Vacations		Vacant
September	R	Wound mgt. [#2.1]	
October			Charting (I) [#6]
November		Discharge interview [#3, #4]	
December	R Holidays		Accreditation readiness

Notes:	R	=	Report to QA committee due
	NCP	=	Nursing care plan
	0	=	Not related to a principal function
	Qu	=	Questionnaire

Exhibit 4.10

QA Calendar — 1992

Mo.	Workload	Audits or Focussed Studies	Clients/Indicators/ Experts
Jan.	Budget		(I) Annual report on Contin. Edn. [#5]
Feb.		Audit of performance appraisals filed in 1991 [#5]	
Mar.			(I) Analysis of deficiencies in manual cheques [#2]++
Apr.		Audit of recruitment function [#1]	
May			(C) Survey of dept. hds. re: HR assistance with Labour Relations [#3]
June		Needs analysis — Staff & mgt. education [#5]+	
July	Vacations		(X) Report on Ministry of Labour visit [#4]
Aug.	Vacations		(I) Analysis of grievances & their disposition [#3]
Sept.			(I) Analysis of late filings with WCB [#2]
Oct.		Audit of personnel policies as meeting legislation [#4]	
Nov.			(C) Analysis of exit interviews 10/91-9/92 [#1]
Dec.	Vacations		Accreditation Readiness survey [#0]

1 = Recruitment (Apr., Nov.)   4 = Personnel policy adm. (July, Oct.)
2 = Salary & benefit adm.(July, Oct.)   5 = Employee services (Jan., Feb., June)
3 = Labour relations (May, Aug.)   0 = Comprehensive review (Dec.)
+   OR Audit of mgt. implementation of 1 collective agreement [#3]
++ OR Analysis of sick time [#2]

References

1. *Collins Dictionary of the English Language* (1986), ed. P. Hanks. Second ed. London: Collins.
2. See, for example, Ontario Hospital Association and Ontario Medical Association (1982). *The Patient Care Appraisal Handbook*. Toronto: OHA.
3. Department of Health (1989). *Working for Patients*. London: HMSO.
4. Goldfield, N. and Nash, D.B., eds. (1989). *Providing Quality Care: The Challenge to Clinicians*. Philadelphia: American College of Physicians, p. 69. See also Chapter 2, "The Patient's Role in Health Care and Quality Assessment," pp. 25-68.
5. *Accreditation Manual for Hospitals* (1992), pp. 103-105.
6. McIver, S. (1991). *An Introduction to Obtaining the Views of Users of Health Services*. London: King's Fund Centre, p. 40.
7. *Ibid.*
8. Weisman, E. and Koch, N., eds. (1989). Patient Satisfaction: *Quality Review Bulletin (QRB) Special Issue15* (6 [June]). See also: Nelson, E.C. *et al.* (1991). The patient comment card: A system to gather customer feedback. *QRB 17* (9 [Sept.]):278-256.
9. Report (1991). Companies grapple with design and response rates in satisfaction surveys. *The Service Edge 4* (5 [May]):2.
10. Petersen, M.B.H. (1989). Using patient satisfaction data: An ongoing dialogue to solicit feedback. *QRB 15* (6 [June]):168.
11. Report, *op. cit.* (see Note 9).
12. Steiber, S.R. and Krowinski, W.J. (1990). *Measuring and Managing Patient Satisfaction*. Chicago: American Hospital Association, p.18.
13. Cunningham, L. (1991). *The Quality Connection in Health Care: Integrating Patient Satisfaction and Risk Management*. San Francisco: Jossey-Bass, pp.143-144.
14. Wilson, C.R.M. (1987). *Hospital-wide Quality Assurance*. Toronto: W.B. Saunders, pp. 56-59.

Part 2

Medical Quality Assurance

5

A Definition of Medical Quality Assurance

5.1
Dr. Codman's
Legacy

Many recent writers[1] begin their account of quality assurance
and medical care quality with the name of E.A. Codman.
Ernest Amory Codman was a surgeon practising in Boston
in the early decades of this century. Out of his own interest
and conscience he kept a record of the operations he
performed and of their outcomes. His "end-result system"
included a retrospective review of the outcomes of each of
his surgery patients one year following the operation.[2] As a
founding member of the American College of Surgeons,
Codman was able in 1914 to gain the College's adoption of
his end-result system. As one of its requirements for
fellowship, each candidate had to submit an abstract of at
least fifty consecutive major operations he had performed,

containing "comprehensive detailed reports on the procedures used, any complications resulting, the elapsed time of the operation and every aspect of the patient's condition."[3]

But for Codman, medical quality was more than just the competence or outcomes of the individual surgeon. He was aware of the important influence on professional behaviour exercised both by major hospitals and by their organized medical staffs. He reported to the Philadelphia County Medical Society how

> *the surgical staff of the Massachusetts General Hospital had reorganized in such a way that each active member of the staff undertook to give special study to some difficult class of cases, and in return the hospital assigned to each member all the cases of that group. The result has been that the mortality in these groups of cases showed a great improvement, and our community has at its service a few men qualified to do each of these difficult operations.*[4]

Codman's concerns were not limited to his profession alone. In his paper "The Product of a Hospital" (1914) he listed fourteen "products of the Massachusetts General Hospital, 1912," including:

> 1. *The results to the 6896 patients*
>
> *Administration:*
> 2. *6896 patients treated*
> 3. *$300 per patient per day*
> 4. *16 days' average stay*
> 5. *320 beds; each bed served 22 patients*
>   *
> *[Under "Education", Codman listed six items; under "Important By-products", he listed two.]*
>   *
> 14. *Important ideas demonstrated*[5]

If individual surgeons should be accountable for the outcomes of their treatment, no less should be expected of hospitals. Codman concluded:

We must formulate some method of hospital report showing as nearly as possible what are the results of the treatment obtained at different institutions. This report must be made out and published by each hospital in a uniform manner so that comparisons will be possible. With such a report as a starting-point those interested can begin to ask questions as to management and efficiency.[6]

In a footnote, Codman reported on the use of what he called "waste products" — wound sepsis, surgical delays, and complications — *outcome indicators,* in today's terminology:

The Massachusetts Hospital has answered these questions by establishing an end-result catalogue. By means of this catalogue and two hours a week, a superintendent, a trustee, or a senior surgeon can keep himself accurately informed as to what is happening to 6000 cases a year.[7]

But Codman was not popular. His demands for peer review, accountability for results, and practice limited by competence were too much for his colleagues. According to contemporary authors,[8] he was forced to leave MGH. He may have been addressing his critics when he wrote:

I am called eccentric for saying in public:
 That hospitals, if they wish to be sure of improvement, must find out what their results are;
 Must analyze their results, to find their strong and weak points;
 Must compare their results with those of other hospitals;
 Must care for what cases they can care for well, and avoid attempting to care for cases which they are not qualified to care for well;
 Must assign the cases to members of the staff [for treatment] for better reasons than seniority, the calendar, or temporary convenience;
 Must welcome publicity not only for their successes, but for their errors, so that the public may give them their help when it is needed;

> *Must promote members of the staff on a basis which
> gives due consideration to what they can and do accomplish
> for their patient.
> Such opinions will not be eccentric a few years hence.*[9]

Once again it was the American College of Surgeons that
endorsed Codman's opinions by adopting them as its own.
He chaired its committee on hospital standardization, whose
Minimum Standard issued in 1917 codified what Codman
had been urging in respect of a hospital's corporate
responsibility for the quality of care. One year later, the
College began its on-site inspection of hospitals to rate their
compliance with its Minimum Standard. This inspection was
the famous Hospital Standardization Program which the
ACS operated until 1951; it was the first hospital accreditation
program in North America and the immediate precursor of
both the current accreditation programs offered in Canada
by CCHFA and in the United States by the Joint Commission
on the Accreditation of Health Care Organizations.

I have a number of reasons for beginning this chapter on
medical quality assurance with Codman and the American
College of Surgeons. First of all, in 1992 — certainly in
Ontario — I find medical staffs alienated by quality
assurance, which too many physicians view as foreign to
medicine and unsympathetic to their practice. It may surprise
them, as this story of Codman surprised me, to discover that
the originators of quality assessment were physicians.
Medical leadership in accreditation has continued to this day
in the United States, and through 1986 in Canada. Second,
Dr. Codman's story well illustrates a continuing feature of
medical QA: it will always remain on the ethical edge of
medical practice, vulnerable to unpopularity, misunder-
standing and pressure. Third, medical QA is more complex
than the PIER model; it has features all its own which were
first stated by Codman and the American College of
Surgeons and which need to be factored into any modern
definition and appraisal of medical care quality. It is to these
that we turn next.

5.2
The Four-Legged
Table

The Minimum Standard, c. 1920

The Minimum Standard against which general hospitals in
the United States and Canada were surveyed in the 1920s by
the American College of Surgeons consisted of five
requirements:

1. *That physicians and surgeons privileged to practice in
   the hospital be organized as a definite group or staff.*

2. *That membership upon the staff be restricted to
   physicians and surgeons who are (a) full graduates of
   medicine in good standing and legally licensed to
   practice in their respective states or provinces, (b)
   competent in their respective fields, and (c) worthy in
   character and in matters of professional ethics; that in
   this latter connection the practice of the division of fees,
   under any guise whatever, be prohibited.*

3. *That the staff initiate and, with the approval of the
   governing board of the hospital, adopt rules,
   regulations, and policies governing the professional
   work of the hospital; that these rules, regulations, and
   policies specifically provide: (a) That staff meetings be
   held at least once each month. . . (b) That the staff
   review and analyze at regular intervals their clinical
   experience in the various departments of the hospital. . . ,
   the clinical records of patients, free and pay, to be the
   basis for such review and analyses.*

4. *That accurate and complete records be written for all
   patients and filed in a manner accessible to the
   hospital. . . .*

> 5. *That diagnostic and therapeutic facilities under*
> *competent supervision be available for the study,*
> *diagnosis, and treatment of patients. . . .*[10]

In spite of its numbering, the Minimum Standard calls for seven elements now distinguished by common usage:

(a) Medical staff organization

(b) Credentials

(c) Regulation of professional practice

(d) Staff participation

(e) Clinical care appraisal

(f) Completion of patient records

(g) Professional supervision of diagnostic facilities

After 1600 surveys carried out by the College, its Dr. Slobe wrote about the early application of the Minimum Standard to hospitals. He commented briefly on five,[11] which had aroused the most difficulty in interpretation:

[On medical staff organization]
There is no standard type of staff organization applicable to all hospitals. . . . There should be, however, a definite organization, including the formation of sufficient committees to cover the various activities of the hospital, in order that responsibility for these activities be accurately centralized.

[On staff participation]
Even though ["courtesy" staff] use the hospital at infrequent intervals, they should be expected to live up to all the obligations which the hospital expects of its regular staff. . . . they are a part of the hospital so long as they send any of their patients there, and. . . they are expected to attend the staff meetings.

[On clinical care appraisal]
The analysis of hospital results is one of the chief objectives of the standardization program. . . . It is the feeling of the College that a large part of the monthly staff meeting should be devoted to an analysis of the casualties including deaths, infections, complications, unimproved cases and, in fact, anything closely related to the clinical work in the hospital.

[On medical records]
Relative to case records, the hospital is the logical repository for the medical history of a community. . . . A very common deficiency in hospitals which have recently instituted record systems is a very brief, stereotyped form of care record which seems to fit about 80 per cent of the patients and gives one very little knowledge of the diagnosis.

The author's final comments concerned the provision and medical supervision of laboratory and radiology facilities. These need not concern us.

The 1972 Standards in Canada

The 1972 *Guide of the Canadian Council on Hospital Accreditation* along with its predecessor, the 1971 *Standards* of the Joint Commission in the United States, were the first substantial departure from the Minimum Standard of the American College of Surgeons which had been the accreditation canon from 1918 to 1951. After five years of work, the Joint Commission moved the basis of its accreditation "from their present level of minimum essential to the level of optimum achievable."[12] How did the Minimum Standard of medical staff organization and practice survive this major revision?

The 1972 *Guide to Hospital Accreditation* prescribes the following principle for the medical staff:

There shall be an organized medical staff that has the overall responsibility for the quality of all medical care provided to patients, and for the ethical conduct and professional practices of its members as well as for accounting therefore to the governing body.[13]

This principle is elucidated in seven Standards, shown in Exhibit 5.1.

(a) *Medical staff organization* is the focus of Standard II in which the election of officers, the establishment of clinical departments and the role of the executive or Medical Advisory Committee (MAC) are outlined. The topic is revisited in Standard VII, which requires the medical staff to develop and adopt, subject to the hospital's governing body, by-laws, rules and regulations.

(b) *Medical staff membership* is addressed in Standard I, the categories of membership in Standard II, and the appointments process in Standard III.

(c) *Professional standards* development and maintenance are required through the actions of what today are called MAC subcommittees: Pharmacy & Therapeutics, Medical Records, Infection Control, Disaster & Emergency, and the Joint Conference committee.

(d) *Physician participation* in medical staff activities is prescribed in three Standards: IV, dealing with committees; V, requiring monthly meetings of clinical departments; and VII, requiring the provision of continuing medical education (CME).

(e) *Medical care evaluation* is the central topic of Standard III. Peer review methods are prescribed for tissue review, the analysis of deaths, and review of infections and complications.[14] Utilization review is identified as a necessary component of medical care evaluation.[15]

Exhibit 5.1
Medical Staff Standards 1972

Standard I — Requirements for Membership and Privileges

Each member of the medical staff shall be qualified for membership, and for the performance of the clinical privileges granted to him.

Standard II — Organization of Medical Staff

The medical staff shall be organized to accomplish its required functions; it shall provide for the election or appointment of its officers, executive and other committees, department heads and/or service chiefs.

Standard III — Evaluation of Professional Qualifications and Performance

The medical staff organization shall strive to create and maintain an optimal level of professional performance of its members through the appointment procedures, the delineation of medical staff privileges and the continual review and evaluation of each member's clinical activities.

Standard IV — Functions Relating to Patient Care

The medical staff shall participate in the development and maintenance of high professional standards by representation on committees concerned with patient care.

Standard V — Medical Staff Meetings

There shall be regular medical staff and departmental meetings to review the clinical work of members, and to complete medical staff administrative duties.

Standard VI — Program of Continuing Professional Education

The medical staff shall provide a continuing program of professional education, or give evidence of participation in such a program.

Standard VII — By-laws, Rules and Regulations

The medical staff shall develop and adopt by-laws, rules and regulations subject to the approval of the governing body, to establish a framework for self-government and a means of accountability to the governing body.

— Canadian Council on Hospital Accreditation (1972). *Guide to Hospital Accreditation, 1972.* Toronto: CCHA

The 1986 Medical Services Standards

There is also a direct line between six of the seven demands of the Minimum Standard and the definition of medical quality assurance in the 1986 accreditation *Standards* in Canada. The 1986 *Standards* [16] were the last ones published before the adoption of a generic format by CCHFA in 1991. Today the wording of the QA Standard for Medical Services is almost identical to that for any hospital department, such as Materials Management.

The QA Standard (VIII), approved by CCHFA in May 1986, requires that "the Medical Staff shall develop and approve a program designed to evaluate the quality of its services." Clause 1 describes the character of the program, Clause 2 the content, and Clause 3 additional elements required of QA programs for teaching units. Clause 2 is a list of nineteen "activities related to the entire medical staff" and five "departmental quality assurance activities." These lists are presented in Exhibit 5.2, in which they are matched with the six essential elements of the Minimum Standard: (a) medical staff organization, (b) credentials and privileges, (c) regulation and surveillance of professional practice or quality control, (d) participation of members in medical staff meetings, (e) clinical care appraisal, and (f) medical records.

Of twenty-four activities, only three are found not to fit easily under these headings. The development of a physician manpower plan and utilization review are activities of the 1980s and 1990s. Both are related to QA: UR is accorded Chapter 7 in this text and human resource planning, particularly in its recruitment element, is intended to sustain the clinical viability of a staff. The third entry, "representation at the level of the governing body" or physician advocacy, is more difficult to relate to the quality of medical care, important though it is to the direction and governance of the hospital.

Exhibit 5.2
QA Activities in the 1986 Accreditation Standards Related to Historic Elements of Medical QA

		Med. Staff Org.	Cred- entials	Med. QC	Staff Meet -ings	Med. Care Appr.	Med. Rec.
1.1	Credentialling		x				
1.2	Review of privileges		x				
1.3	MD manpower plan						
1.4	Bylaws, rules, regulationss			x			
1.5	MD participation				x	x	
1.6	Utilization review						
1.7	Representation on board						
1.8	Selection of dept. heads	x					
1.9	Med. staff committees	x					
1.10	MAC subcommittee activity	x					
1.11	Med. staff meetings				x		
1.12	• Review of statistics			x			
	• Criteria audits					x	
	• Clinical records review			x		x	x
	• Tissue review			x			
	• M&M review*			x			
	• Autopsies			x			
	• Complications			x			
	• Complaints			x			
2.3	Departmental activities						
	• Case presentations					x	
	• Organized rounds				x		
	• M&M review*			x			
	• Business meeting	x					
	• Criteria review					x	

* Mortality & Morbidity review

The Analogy of a Table

The title of this section, "The Four-Legged Table," is intended as an analogy for medical quality assurance. The tabletop is labelled "medical staff organization for quality of care." Its four legs are (1) membership or credentialling, (2) physician participation, (3) regulation of practice and quality control, and (4) medical care appraisal. The table analogy is intended both to itemize the essential components of medical quality assurance (see Exhibit 5.3) and to demonstrate their inseparable relationship: without its top the legs would tumble; without its legs the top would be but a side of wood. Each of these is discussed in sections 5.3 through 5.7, which follow. Consolidated reporting occupies section 5.8.

Exhibit 5.3
Medical QA as a Four-Legged Table

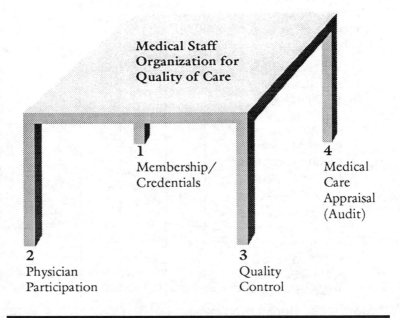

Medical Staff Organization for Quality of Care

1 Membership/ Credentials

4 Medical Care Appraisal (Audit)

2 Physician Participation

3 Quality Control

5.3
Leg #1:
Membership —
Medical
Credentials

If there were a means of securing the services of only the best family physicians, surgeons, paediatricians, obstetricians and others, this would be a hospital's premier assurance of quality of medical care. Second, it would be important to ensure that each physician perform within the range of competence established by his or her specialty and training. Third, it would be ideal if physicians were to practise their skills, and keep them current, by participating in events that ensure that they remain conversant with the continuing evolution of medical science and practice. These are the three essentials of medical credentialling: the screening of initial applications, the delineation of privileges, and the handling of reappointments.

The topic of medical credentialling has been well presented in several U.S. texts recently, written for the profession[17] and the lay trustee.[18] Although the four texts I have cited (see References at the end of this chapter) are American and thus are based upon different laws and the employment of a national practitioner data bank, their descriptions of the credentialling process and the roles of medical staff and boards of trustees are generally reliable from a Canadian standpoint. In addition, it is generally conceded that Canadian hospitals handle initial applications reliably and appropriately and the delineation of privileges quite effectively. Accordingly, this section will be problem oriented and deal with two issues: reappointments, and credentialling in small hospitals. In discussing these topics we shall deal in risk management as much as in quality assurance. The securing of excellent practitioners and the avoidance of those who are incompetent are just two sides of the same coin.

The Handling of Reapplications

Public hospitals acts in Canada say that medical staff appointments can be made for only one year, although they continue in force until reappointments are made or denied in the following year. The necessity for annual reappointment — in the U.S. medical appointments last for two years — has created an annual ritual in many Canadian hospitals. In the fall of each year the credentials committee takes out their 200, 50 or 10 physician files, leafs through them, and unless their attention is grabbed by a notice of suit, a disciplinary letter from the Chief or a letter from the College of Physicians and Surgeons, recommends to the Medical Advisory Committee the reappointment of all 200, 50 or 10 physicians. The MAC concurs in a fifteen-second vote. The Chief of Staff then takes the MAC's recommendation to the board, which concurs with similar alacrity. The function follows the law, not the law's intent.

The law recognizes that the right to treat should be restricted to those who maintain their clinical competence and should not be automatically granted forever to those who qualified once in the past. If credentialling is viewed as an essential element in quality assurance, then a medical staff must find ways to move beyond the ritual of the law and to re-establish its intent. Two procedures merit consideration: the use of cohorts, and the institution of a triennial review.

Reappointment in Cohorts

In spite of having two-year tenure for medical appointments, U.S. hospitals commonly divide their staffs into cohorts for reappointment purposes. This allows their credentials committees to consider and recommend reappointments quarterly in respect of one cohort — one-eighth of the staff — at a time. This simple strategy should appeal to all three parties involved in the credentialling process: management, the MAC, and the board. Instead of the December ritual at which all staff are reappointed by acclamation, under the cohort system, physicians would be reappointed by name in

December, March, June or September. As credentials
committees have to meet throughout the year to consider
new applications and locums, some staffs arrange their
reappointment load in as many cohorts as they have
meetings per year (nine or ten).

Proposal: A Triennial Review

With a physician's credentials under review every twelve
months, it is unrealistic to expect that a credentials
committee will either see the need or have the time to carry
out a special or detailed review of any doctor unless alerted
by special circumstances, or negative indicators. A better
alternative might be a detailed review of the credentials of
each physician every third year from the date of his or her
initial appointment. The intent here is to go beyond the
signatures on the reapplication form and ask questions of his
or her performance in three respects:

- The physician's actual use of the treatment privileges on
  his or her list;

- The physician's clinical outcomes, as represented by
  length of stay, incidents and adverse patient occurrences;
  and

- Evidence of continuing medical education (CME)
  through attendance at CME sessions, and participation in
  medical staff committees and clinical audit activities.

Each medical staff will carry out this kind of review in its
own manner, incidentally negotiated with the staff. A minimum
requirement must be the perusal of Hospital Medical Records
Institute (HMRI) data comparing the physician's performance
either with matched cases or, when possible, with his or her
professional peers on staff, in respect of principal procedures
or most important case-mix groups (CMGs).

In the course of these triennial reviews, credentials
committees have two responsibilities: to note changes in
physician performance and to determine the appropriateness
of the applicants' privilege list. The maxim "Use them or

lose them" should be the rule with respect to privileges, and few reviews should conclude without recommendations for changes in a physician's list. Triennial reviews can be justified *only* if undertaken in conjunction with the continuous monitoring of outcome indicators and performance standards by the MAC or clinical departments.

Credentialling in Small Hospitals

Small medical staffs have two major problems in maintaining a conscientious credentialling process. Small staffs know their members too well either to be objective or to make recommendations without the possibility of conflict of interest. Second, there is often no professional peer for some specialists on staff, such as the hospital's only surgeon, internist or psychiatrist.

I have for some years recommended that hospitals commission an external physician review of their specialty areas — Emergency, Labour & Delivery, the Operating Suite — from the most appropriate or accessible teaching hospital. I am indebted to lawyer Joshua Liswood[19] for the idea of incorporating such an outside specialist into the credentialling process. Under Liswood's scheme, the credentials committee would refer a dozen or so recent charts of the staff member for review by a chosen specialist in a teaching hospital, and make its recommendations based on the specialist's advice. Why should a lawyer give this kind of advice? Because a lawyer recognizes the hospital's vulnerability to the allegation that its credentialling process is incompetent, in the absence of peers, to assess its specialists.

While Liswood's suggestion does not address the issue of overfamiliarity, there is a practical solution available to small staffs. Some small hospitals have their regional medical centre do their credentialling for them. Alternatively, small staffs might combine their credentialling function with that of their closest hospital(s). A joint committee of two to four members will be able to show more objectivity than a small staff acting on its own.

5.4
Leg #2:
Participation

As a layman learning about medical staff affairs, I could not understand those who took physicians to task for resisting mandatory attendance at medical staff or department meetings. It seemed to me that physicians shared my own estimation of the overproliferation of meetings and committees encumbering the work of many hospitals. Only recently have I come to appreciate the importance of physician participation in the life of the organized medical staff. Physicians are the only professional group in the hospital bound by their own by-laws, rules and regulations. The fact that they work within the hospital but are not employed by it only partially explains the rules on their attendance. Solo decision-making and solo practice are inherent to medicine. While physicians will call for tests, confer with radiologists and pathologists, discuss cases with their colleagues and call formally for consultations, they expect to be in charge of their cases and take sole responsibility for them. Threats to their autonomy, whether from hospital staff or medical colleagues, are dealt with summarily. Mandatory attendance at meetings and the annual requirement to sign off on the Public Hospitals Act, the hospital by-laws and medical staff rules, have to be understood in the context of the physician's (laudable) obsession with his or her own practice and consequent tendency to isolationism.

The demand that doctors attend meetings and otherwise participate in medical staff activities has been heard since the 1920s. The question physicians most commonly raise is, to what ends? I can suggest four. First, the medical staff and its activities will be strengthened by virtue of full participation. Often the weakness of medical QA can be traced to the fact that it is a minority activity. While it is pursued by the conscientious, it fails to engage or review the sloppy or the driven — both of whom can make major errors.

Second, participation and attendance aids in professional communication among a group whose solo practice makes communication naturally difficult. The clinical care given by all members is enhanced by their myriad informal conversations over meals, in corridors, and before and after meetings.

Third, affiliation with the medical staff of a respected hospital influences individual practice. Although Codman was writing in medicine's pre-professional days, his advice is still valid:

> *Great institutions are checks on the frailties of human nature. . . . The great surgeon or physician may be avaricious, mean, ill-natured at home, jealous, even immoral or drunken; but when he appears for public duty at the hospital he must at least assume the appearance of virtue and efficiency. . . . in the public institution the trained watchful eyes of his assistants, consultants, and nurses are ever on him. . . . To hold his position he must travel and read, at least somewhat, to keep up appearances, and the habit of self-examination thus formed reacts on his private practice.*[20]

A number of recent studies have demonstrated that one of the key variables in determining quality of medical care is the strength of the physician's affiliation with the hospital whose care was being studied.[21] In at least one study,[22] strength of affiliation was a stronger determinant than the physician's formal training or clinical experience.

Fourth, physician participation helps to determine the quality of the medical staff and its corporate conduct. Quality of care and ethical values are the possession not of individual practitioners but of the entire staff — or at least of particular departments. Further, medical staffs get the leaders they are prepared to live with: a keen staff will get a keen Chief; a commercial staff will find an accommodating Chief. Although hospitals may be governed by the same Public Hospitals Act and physicians by essentially the same by-laws, rules and regulations, the corporate culture of one medical staff can promote high quality, excellent interprofessional relations, and strong participation in hospital affairs, while that of another can fall prey to elitism, factionalism, and the avoidance of corporate responsibility.

5.5
Leg #3:
Quality Control

I am indebted to Kenneth Williams [23] for the realization that quality control is alive and not dead and is an essential function of the organized medical staff. Williams distinguishes quality control from medical care appraisal, and has thus enabled me to make the same distinction and to appreciate QC's continuing importance. Quality control has to do with the regulation of professional practice or, to quote the Minimum Standard, the demand "that the staff initiate. . . and adopt rules, regulations, and policies governing the professional work of the hospital."[24]

Among the rules specified were those for monthly staff meetings and the analysis of clinical experience. The separation between quality control, which is the regular inspection of data to see that clinical standards are being met, and medical care appraisal, which is the topic-focussed audit or other inquiry, probably occurred with the 1977 accreditation *Standards* in Canada. At that time clinical standards became the property of the medical staff and were monitored by its committees, whereas patient care appraisal was taken up by medical departments. Readers can refer to Standards IV and V in Exhibit 5.1 (page 123). The same distinction is carried in the 1986 *Standards,* where the following items are listed[25] as the minimum agenda for departmental meetings:

- Case presentation

Exhibit 5.4
Common Indicators Monitored by Five Standing Subcommittees of the MAC

1. Tissue & Audit

Deaths, all in-patient deaths, deaths within 48 h of surgery

Autopsy rate

Transfers to other hospitals (higher level of care)

Complications, surgical and medical

Unimproved cases

Surgical cases with minimal pathology

Appendectomies, T&As

Blood transfusion reactions; single-unit transfusions

Discrepancies in diagnosis, pre-op and post-op

Obstetrical Indicators:

Operations on reproductive organs

Abortions

Caesarean section rate

Obstetrical anaesthesia

Deliveries without an MD in attendance

2. Medical Records

Incomplete charts:

- Number for signature only
- Number for completion

Records:

- Without history and physical within 72 h
- Without adequate progress notes

Failure to record pre-operative diagnosis before surgery

Problems with patient consent: missing, discrepant (i.e., lack of concurrence between consent and intervention)

3. Utilization

Audit of long-stay cases
Cancellations and postponements
Emergency and urgent admissions
Transfers to extended-care facilities
Inappropriate in-patient placements
Radiology (and/or Laboratory) on-call hours and call-backs
The following statistics are often reviewed routinely:
Operations, consultation rates
Laboratory units, radiology examinations, physiotherapy attendances
Referrals to home care program, pre-admission testing
Monthly costs of medical-surgical supplies,
Occupancy, patient days, average length of stay

4. Pharmacy & Therapeutics

Adverse drug reactions
Medication incidents
Changes to hospital formulary: Additions and deletions
Non-formulary drugs ordered
Poly-pharmacy: Drugs per patient

5. Infection Control

Infectious admissions
Nosocomial infections
Postoperative wound infections
Urinary tract infections
Gastrointestinal/ *E.coli* infections

Infections by type:

Viral, parasitic/fungal, other non-bacterial, Legionella and other
environmental, STDs including AIDS, TB.

Preventive measures:

Vaccination programs, by patient and type
Disposal of sharps, incidents
Catheter care

- Organized and recorded rounds
- Reviews of morbidity and mortality
- Business meetings
- Reviews of medical care based on established criteria

Medical staffs establish their own committees, which are subcommittees of the Medical Advisory Committee. Most of them are named in the medical staff by-laws with terms of reference, and are thus standing committees. Those named in the 1990 *OHA/OMA Prototype Hospital By-laws*[26] include: Credentials, Medical Records, Medical Quality Assurance, Infection Control, Utilization, and Pharmacy & Therapeutics. Some staffs have an Education committee, and most will probably prefer their historic Tissue & Audit committee to one labelled QA. Three aspects of committees deserve note: first, they belong and report to the MAC. Second, their mandate runs across all departments. Third, they deal with medical staff standards. Committees will take generic problems back to the MAC, whereas specific problems will be referred to the Chief of Staff or a department chief.

Rather than discuss the types of monitoring systems and standards adopted by committees, I have developed lists for each of five committees, omitting Credentials and preferring Tissue & Audit to Medical QA (see Exhibit 5.4). The essential conclusion, however, is that notwithstanding QA, CQI/TQM, or any other inspired excellence system devised in the future, a medical staff will always need to maintain its quality control function. QC is as much a defence for the practitioner as for the patient, and should provide a fail-safe system for both. It is the foundation of medical risk management.

5.6
Leg #4: Medical
Care Appraisal

Of the four components of medical QA, this was probably
the last to be developed, beginning with Codman's
retrospective case review. Its development has been greatly
aided by the development of standards for the completion
and data processing of health records. Medical scholarship
and research has also played its part in isolating the questions
that can be asked of medical care and in developing the
means of inquiry. It was formally introduced as a distinct
element in medical quality assurance by the Joint
Commission in its 1976 *Standards,* complete with quotas on
the number of audits to be undertaken per year. In 1979 the
Joint Commission abolished quotas and changed the
emphasis from the volume of audits to their ability to solve
perceived problems. In Canada, CCHA followed the Joint
Commission; medical audit appeared in its *Standards* in
1977, and problem solving was the definition of quality
assurance when it was first introduced in 1983. In both
jurisdictions, JCAH's 1975 publication of the *Performance
Evaluation Procedure for Auditing and Improving Patient
Care* caused medical audit to eclipse the other methods of
clinical evaluation, particularly those carried out by medical
staff committees. It tended also to be seen as the only form
of medical care appraisal.[27] Both of these misunderstandings
have needed to be addressed.

Performance Evaluation Procedure provided a practical,
step-by-step guide to what was then a new discipline, as did
other texts in Canada some years later. Exhibit 5.5
summarizes the seven steps advocated by the OHA and OMA
in their 1982 *Patient Care Appraisal Handbook.* The topic of
patient care appraisal is treated in practical terms both in
Chapter 4 ("The Assessment of Professional Performance")
and Chapter 6 ("Medical Care Appraisal") of this text.

Exhibit 5.5

Procedure for Medical Audit: Seven Steps Common to Most Review Studies

1. Choose a topic

2. Set objectives

3. Establish the criteria

4. Retrieve the data

5. Collate and present the results of the study

6. Analyze by peer review, and report

7. Take action and follow up.

— Ontario Hospital Association/Ontario Medical Association (1982). *Patient Care Appraisal Handbook*. Toronto: OHA/OMA, p. 24. Reproduced with permission.

Recent literature points to a move away from medical audit on the part of both the Canadian and U.S. accreditation bodies. In 1986 the JCAHO published a guide on monitoring care through the use of performance indicators.[28] (See "Monitoring and Evaluation Process" on page 175 of this text.) But the future of medical audit is made more uncertain by the endorsement of continuous quality improvement by both bodies, beginning with their 1991 accreditation *Standards.*

As Chapter 6 discusses medical care appraisal, there is little need to say more here. Clinical care appraisal should be seen as one of four contributors to the quality of medical care, and one of four fruits of an effective medical staff organization.

5.7
The Medical Staff Organization

From time to time across Canada, the provincial hospital (health care) associations and medical associations, often in conjunction with the provincial ministry of health, issue prototype hospital by-laws. The first section (#61) of the Ontario Medical Staff By-laws (1990 edition) reads:

> *Purpose of the Medical Staff Organization*
> *The purposes of the medical staff organization. . . are: to provide a structure whereby the members of the medical staff participate in the Hospital's planning, policy setting, and decision making, and to serve as a quality assurance system for medical care rendered to patients by the medical staff and to ensure the continuing improvement of the quality of medical care.*[29]

This statement expresses perfectly the inherent duality with both the medical staff organization and the physician's practice. Physicians are at one and the same time entrepreneurs and care givers. The former role is expressed through the elective processes of the medical staff, whose officers sit on the hospital board. The latter is seen in the authority delegated by the board to the Chief of Staff, chiefs of department and Medical Advisory Committee. This duality occurs at the personal level in the physician's use of time, and the tension between the corporate demands and the insistent demands of "my" practice. We will need to return to this tension with reference to QA participation later.

The medical staff organization is both the result of credentialling, participation, quality control and medical care appraisal, and what makes them happen. Its essentials are individual *leadership*, widely shared *responsibility*, and meaningful *activity*. These form a triangle, as each depends on the other two. Without leadership, medical staff activity deteriorates into the conduct of rituals required by law and custom. Without the sharing of responsibility, medical staff activity becomes a minority occupation; its leadership tires and loses respect. Meaningful activity hooks the individual, claiming his or her time, interest and involvement; it leads the individual to seek change and push for improvement. This person in turn becomes a leader, as he or she shares responsibility and later is recognized by appointment to office. All the while, time and the claims of practice pull at the uninvolved, deplete attendance at committees that have lost their direction, and create reluctance to get involved.

Effective medical staff organization depends on the felicitous choice of a Chief of Staff by the board with the advice of medical staff, and the election of strong chiefs of department on the basis of their clinical competence, ethical practice, interpersonal skills and leadership ability. The second requisite is a limited number of MAC subcommittees, each with clear terms of reference and good expertise. The third requirement is a contributory role in the organization for all active staff. This last will be impossible in larger hospitals, but a target to be aimed for in those with organized departments and fewer than 100 active staff. Roles should be found for all staff within their departments, or on MAC committees, *ad hoc* committees or audit teams — all of them with meaningful tasks.

In *Medical Staff Peer Review*, D.A. Lang identifies eight key expectations of physicians joining a medical staff.

> *By meeting these eight expectations, the individual will perceive value in the group relationship. Value will lead to defense of group processes and standards, despite personal cost. For the group, then, understanding and meeting these expectations is its reason for being. The group must be aware of the expectations of its members in all actions it takes.*[30]

Dr. Lang's list,[31] which is not rank-ordered, includes:

- *Professional autonomy.* "The core value of the physician is his or her autonomy as a professional."

- *Control of quality.* "The new physician is entitled to expect that the medical staff will have in place an effective program for the monitoring of quality."

- *Patient advocacy.* "The physician has the unique responsibility for determining the special patient needs and managing the system so they are met."

- *Peer reliability.* ". . . provides a sense of security to the novice physician, leading to a sense of esprit and confidence in the group."

- *Fair process.* "Given the right of the medical staff to take corrective action that can deprive the physician of civil and professional rights, as well as livelihood, there is an accompanying obligation for fair processes."

- *Equal access.* "The individual physician is entitled to expect a fair and explicit system for the allocation of beds for patients and time for procedures."

- *Access to information.* "A structured program of academic information, updating [clinical] knowledge. . . . Departmental communication of quality assurance and peer review experience. . . . Regular hospital market analysis."

- *Consistency of hospital services.* "The individual physician expects that the hospital will respond accurately and consistently to a patient's identified needs."

I have permitted myself to borrow extensively from Dr. Lang's excellent guide since I am not a physician, and even if I were to know what physician applicants sought in a medical staff, I would have no authority to describe it. My own work with physicians has convinced me that they believe in exchange relationships, that is, they will invest time and energy in activities that offer them some return or personal value. For this reason, I tend to be less comfortable working with physicians whose sole motivation seems to be altruistic. Altruism is unreliable, and it is unfair to ask people who have important and high-paying responsibilities to engage in activities that do not repay them. The rewards are seldom monetary. Instead personal protection, peer recognition, clinical learning, the satisfaction of having solved a problem or created a better system, or the assurance of a fairer distribution of clinical resources may all be relevant motivations for work on behalf of the group or staff. Dr. Lang's eight benefits are an excellent place to begin an analysis of medical staff organization and effectiveness.

5.8
Rendering
Account

Chiefs of Staff and Vice Presidents of Medicine often find accreditation surveys embarrassing: they may feel that their staffs have not done enough — although no one knows or says what is enough — and they have little idea what it is that CCHFA surveyors will wish to see. Indeed, there is no guidance as to what should be presented. Consequently, the physician surveyors are allowed simply to set off on their own fishing expedition through the staff's incidental documentation: minutes, books, credential files, and current health records chosen at random.

When I was asked to do a pre-accreditation survey in a small hospital, the Chief of Staff raised the question of what he should have ready and what, if anything, he needed to show. Having recognized that medical QA entailed much more than audit and, in fact, having developed the four- or five-component model (depending on whether medical staff organization is distinguished from activity), I designed the form shown in Exhibit 5.6 at the end of this chapter.

Finally, there is a QA Calendar of the sort proposed in Chapter 4, which lists or schedules the three elements: committee activity, performance indicator review, and patient care appraisals. This kind of form fulfills two significant needs for most medical staffs. It provides a method of reporting on the various quality management activities the staff supports, and its questions set some goals and limits for the staff. If I am pushed further on the limits on medical audits per year — and I often am — then I suggest the following:

- Every staff should complete a minimum of four audits per year. Where active staff number fewer than ten to twelve MDs, the minimum can be met by engaging in interdisciplinary or team audits (e.g., in Emergency and Long-Term Care).

- Where staff is departmentalized, each department should complete at least two audits per year, in addition to monitoring its own indicators.

It is more difficult to describe optimal activity, as this will be determined by the size and distribution of each medical staff. However, I believe that every active staff member should take part in an audit, as a member of an audit committee, no less frequently than once in two years. This will pose problems for larger staffs.

But accreditation is not the only occasion on which a medical staff should give account. The format shown in Exhibit 5.6 can also be used by Chiefs of Staff in the preparation of their annual reports to the hospital corporation and the community.

Exhibit 5.6
Format for the Annual Report
of a Hospital Medical Staff

I.   Medical Staff Membership

---

1. Composition

The current (date) composition of the medical staff includes:

Medical Staff Membership

Specialty	1 Active	2 Associate	3 Courtesy	4 *Locum Tenens*	5 Temporary	Totals Actual	PMP*
Family Medicine							
Internal Medicine							
Paediatrics							
Psychiatry							
Surgery							
Anaesthesia							
Obstetrics/ Gynaecology							

*Physician Manpower Plan

2. Recruitment

During the last year a total of _____ physicians have been interviewed/ encouraged to apply for membership. Physicians and management have engaged in the following activities to attract physicians to the hospital and community:

_____

_____

_____

3. The Credentials Committee

3.1 During the course of the year (__ / __ /9__ to __ / __ /9__) the Credentials Committee considered and made recommendations on applications. Of these it:

	Appointments	Reappointments	Totals
Recommended			
Requested more info.			
Did NOT recommend			

3.2 It recommended the following changes from associate to active: _____, and from (status) to (status): _____ .

3.3 It voted to increase _____ members' treatment privileges;

decrease _____ members' treatment privileges,

at the member's request: _____, for cause: _____

_____

_____

3.4 The Credentials Committee processes all annual reappointments at *one* time Yes___ No ___ ,
   or
by cohorts in two ___ three ___ four ___ separate months.

Members' credentials are subject to detailed review every third ___ fourth ___ fifth year.   Yes ___ No ___.

4. **Miscellaneous Activities**

Notes should be made of such activities as:
- Review or revision of the application form
- Review or revision of the definition of treatment privileges
- Opportunities to educate the board on the credentialling process
- Voluntary resignation of appointments by members, on retirement or relocation
- All suspensions, revocations or withdrawals of privileges
- Member appeals against the advice of the Credentials Committee
- Occasions when the advice of the Credentials Committee was rejected by the MAC or the board.

II. Medical Staff Organization and Activity

1. **Leadership**

	Name	Term (19__ - 19__)
Chief of Staff:		
Chief of Emergency:		
President		
Vice President		
Secretary/Treasurer		

2. **Support**

Medical staff activities were assisted by the following staff support from the hospital:

Health records ____ h per week

Secretarial ____ h per week

3. Representation

Medical staff representation on governing and administrative bodies:

Board of Trustees _____

_____

_____

Committees of the Board

Executive _____

Finance _____

Planning _____

_____ _____

_____ _____

Number of Meetings of Joint Conference Committee

this year (199__) _____

last year (199__) _____

_____

4. Medical Staff Activities

	n of Meetings		Attendance	
	This Year	Last Year	This Year	Last Year
4.1 Medical Staff Meetings				
Percentage Attendance				
4.2 Meetings of Organized Departments				
Medicine				
Surgery				
Obstetrics				
Paediatrics				
etc.				

5. Medical Advisory Committee

5.1 Membership

Position	Name
Chief of Staff (Chairman)	
President	
...	
...	

5.2 MAC Subcommittees

Committee	Chair	Members
Credentials		
Tissue & Audit		
Medical Records		
Quality Assurance		
Pharmacy (P&T)		
Utilization		
Infection Control		
Emergency		
Long-Term Care		
etc.		

Number of active and associate members of the medical staff active on MAC and subcommittee: ____ / ____ %

6. Continuing Medical Education (CME)

6.1 CME required in medical staff by-laws or rules:

_____

_____

_____

6.2 Regular CME sessions

Number held ____ Attendance ____

6.3 Special sessions held

Date ____ Topic ____ Faculty/Resource ____ Attendance ____

III. Medical Monitoring

1. Committee Activity

	1992 ˙OND	1993 JFM	1993 AMJ	1993 JAS	Totals
Credentials					
Tissue & Audit					
Medical Records					
Utilization					
QA					
Pharmacy					
Education					
Infection Control					
Emergency					
Long-Term Care					
Disaster					

˙Month of meeting *or* reporting to MAC

2. Quality Control

For each committee, attach a list of monitoring routines and studies carried out in previous year (or 18 months).

3. Performance Indicators

List the performance indicators established by the medical staff to monitor ongoing performance. Where appropriate, the indicator should be linked to its principal function. List the agency (committee, MAC, Chief) that monitors each indicator and the frequency.

IV. Patient Care Appraisal

1. Studies Completed

List, in order of their completion, the various audits and other studies carried out in the last 18 months (this calendar year and the last). For each, provide a one-paragraph summary covering its focus, population, method, findings, and follow-up.

2. Studies Planned and In Progress

List those studies which are planned and/or underway, and enter an identifier for each in column 3 of the QA Calendar, attached.

PF#   Topic   Target Date   Investigator

References

1. See, for example: Graham, N.O. (1982). *Quality Assurance in Hospitals: Strategies for Assessment and Implementation.* Rockville, MD: Aspen, pp. 6-7; Carroll, J.G. (1984). *Restructuring Hospital Quality Assurance: The New Guide for Health Care Providers.* Homewood, IL: Dow-Jones Irwin, pp. 8-9; Eisenberg, J.M. and Kabcenell, A. (1988). Organized practice and the quality of medical care. *Inquiry* 25(Spring):78-79; Goldfield, N. and Nash, D.B. (1989). *Providing Quality Care: The Challenge to Clinicians.* Philadelphia: American College of Physicians, p. 8; Bader, B.S. (1991). *Informing the Board about Quality.* Rockville, MD: Bader & Associates, p. 6; Orlikoff, J.E. and Totten, M.K. (1991). *The Board's Role in Quality Care: A Practical Guide for Hospital Trustees.* Chicago: American Hospital Association, pp. 11-13.
2. Lohr, K.N. (1990). *Medicare: A Strategy for Quality Assurance* (vol. I). Washington, D.C.: National Academy Press, p. 65, note 4.
3. Carroll, *op. cit.* (see Note 1), p. 9.
4. Codman, E.A. (1914). The product of a hospital. *Surgery, Gynaecology & Obstetrics 18*:495.
5. *Ibid.,* p. 496.
6. *Ibid.,* p. 494.
7. *Ibid.,* p. 495.
8. Orlikoff & Totten (see Note 1), p. 12; Eisenberg & Kabcenell (see Note 1), pp. 78-79.
9. Codman, E.A. (1916). *A Study in Hospital Efficiency: The First Five Years.* Boston: Thomas Todd. Quoted in: American Hospital Association (1991). *Practice Pattern Analysis: A Tool for Continuous Improvement of Patient Care.* Chicago: AHA, p. 1.
10. *Bulletin of the American College of Surgeons VII* (4) [January 1924], quoted in: Orlikoff & Totten, *op. cit.,* p.13.
11. Slobe, F.W. (1923). The Minimum Standard and its application to hospitals. *Bulletin of the American College of Surgeons 7*(1):7-9.
12. Canadian Council on Hospital Accreditation (1972). *The Guide to Hospital Accreditation.* Toronto: CCHA, p. vii.
13. *Ibid.,* p. 11.
14. *Ibid.,* p. 19.
15. *Ibid.,* pp. 19-20.

16. Canadian Council on Hospital Accreditation (1986). *Standards for Accreditation of Canadian Health Facilities.* Ottawa: CCHA.
17. Eisele, C.W., Fifer, W.R. and Wilson, T.C. (1985). *The Medical Staff and the Modern Hospital.* Englewood, CO: Estes Park Institute; see also Lang, D.A. (1991). *Medical Staff Peer Review.* Chicago: American Hospital Association.
18. Bader, B.S. (1991). *Informing the Board about Medical Staff Credentialling and Development.* Rockville, MD: Bader & Associates; see also Orlikoff & Totten (1991), *op. cit.* (see Note 1).
19. Liswood, J. of Sawers, Liswood, Scott. Personal communication, Timmins, Ontario 13 February 1992.
20. Codman, *op. cit.* (see Note 4), p. 494.
21. Shortell, S.M. and LoGerfo, J.P. (1981). Hospital medical staff organization and quality of care. *Medical Care* *XIX*(10):1041-1055.
22. Flood, A.B., Scott, W.R., Ewy, W. and Forrest, W.H. Jr. (1982). Effectiveness in professional organizations: The impact of surgeons and surgical staff organizations on quality of care in hospitals. *Health Services Research 17*(4):341-363. See also: Garber, A.M., Fuchs, V.R., and Silverman, J.F. (1984). Case mix, costs, and outcomes: Differences between faculty and community services in a university hospital. *New England Journal of Medicine 310*(19 [May 10]):1231-1237.
23. Personal communication, December 1990. Also see: Williams, K.J. and Donnelly, P.R. (1982). *Medical Care Quality and the Public Trust.* Chicago: Pluribus, pp. 197-209.
24. See Note 10.
25. CCHA, *op. cit.* (see Note 16), Clause 2.2.3, p. 32.
26. The Ontario Hospital Association and the Ontario Medical Association (1990). *Prototype Hospital By-laws.* Toronto: OHA.
27. Affeldt, J.E., Roberts, J.S. and Walczak, R.M. (1983). Quality assurance: Its origin, status, and future direction - A JCAH perspective. *Evaluation and the Health Professions 6*(2):245-255.
28. Joint Commission on the Accreditation of Hospitals (1986). Monitoring and evaluation of the quality and appropriateness of care. *Quality Review Bulletin [QRB] 12*(9 [Sept.]):326-330.
29. OHA, *op. cit.* (see Note 25), p. 38.
30. Lang, *op. cit.* (see Note 17), p. 90.
31. *Ibid.,* pp. 90-96.

6

Medical Care Appraisal

6.1
Getting
Organized

For Quality — Against Quality Assurance

Anyone who listens to medical staff leaders in Ontario might
quickly come to the conclusion that there were two types of
medical quality assurance (QA) programs in hospitals —
those that are moribund and those with problems. If you
were to press the disillusioned chiefs further, you would
likely hear one of two generic descriptions: (1) medical QA is
frantic activity within four to six months of accreditation
survey, with silence before and after; or (2) it is a minority
activity carried out by keeners behind closed doors,
suspected by "real" physicians, and tolerated only if it leaves
them alone. In this sorry situation, the apparent villain is
poor motivation on the part of physicians.

As a non-physician, I am fascinated by this state of affairs. QA and medical practice seem to me to be natural allies. QA was not invented by government regulators, hospital administrators or physiotherapists, but by Dr. E.A. Codman and the American College of Surgeons (see Chapter 5). The medical audit process is akin to clinical research, and peer review to clinical rounds in third- and fourth-year medicine. The surveillance systems provided by ongoing committee activity should afford protection to the individual clinician, not just embarrassment. But the reality is that physicians and QA have become adversaries. How to bridge the gap between them?

Two fallacies in the vexed discussion of MDs and QA need to be identified. The first is that medical QA is synonymous with medical audit. Quality assurance is the term for *all* those means that are used to assure quality — not just one of them. As we saw in Chapter 5, QA and its five components were developed by the medical profession. The exposure of the "medical audit" fallacy has practical importance: it takes the pressure off medical leaders and off audit and peer review. It allows for a re-evaluation of the parts of medical staff activity that are effective, and permits more patience with, and support for, medical audit.

The second fallacy is that, because physicians abhor QA, they are not concerned about quality. This is a destructive *non sequitur.* It is like saying that because a man dislikes New York he hates America. The truth of the matter is that physicians are vitally concerned about the quality of the care *they* give, for reasons both positive (they care about their patients) and negative (the results of poor care are many and all are unpleasant). Physicians change their clinical practices over the course of a year, trying new drugs, techniques and regimens all because of their quest for effectiveness in care — or quality. So the truth about their rejection of QA lies elsewhere. To use a religious analogy: churchgoing in Canada has been declining for more than thirty years. For many people the issue is not that they have lost their faith, but simply that they can no longer express their faith through the historic rituals of the churches. So too with QA: physicians do not find its practices to be quality enhancing.

We will return to physicians' views of QA, but not before looking at the consequences of this insight. If it is allowed that physicians are vitally concerned about the quality of their care but feel estranged from quality assurance, we have exposed a new alternative. Instead of changing physician motivation, it may be easier to change QA so that physicians will find its practices quality enhancing.

Medical Inhibitions and Some Rewards

I asked a group of medical staff leaders from Manitoba hospitals what their hospital colleagues thought about QA. Their answers came out quicker than I could write them on the flip chart:

> *Time. . . . No remuneration. . . . Too busy. . . .*
> *Intimidating and discomforting to assess peers. . . .*
> *Perception of overkill in accountability — already more*
> *than enough systems in place. . . . Apathy. . . . Unrealistic*
> *expectations. . . . Threat of loss of confidentiality. . . . Not*
> *seen as an educational process. . . . Paperwork. . . . Not as*
> *interesting as clinical work. . . . Not as demanding as*
> *clinical work (patient is there, the phone rings). . . .*
> *Uncertainty as to its purpose and value. . . . A form of*
> *policing. . . . No recognition. . . . Boring. . . . Repetitive*
> *(unoriginal routine). . . . Inadequate support systems. . . .*
> *No feedback to MDs. . . . Uncertainty about process. . . .*
> *(Winnipeg, 24 May 1991)*

At the 1991 CAQA Conference, Duane McGregor, a clinician from the Hospital for Sick Children, tried to explain the physician's alienation from QA. She compared the physician's perception with those of QA co-ordinators. Her slide read:

Help us see the positives:

We See	You See
• *More work*	• *Improved efficiency*
• *Bureaucracy*	• *Safer environment for patients*
• *Paper shuffle*	• *Monitoring, identifying problems*
• *Threat of standards/ "cookbook medicine"*	• *Protection against malpractice*

In these and other comments from doctors, I hear at least five distinguishable negative perceptions of medical audit, which many see as synonymous with QA.

The first is *time;* physicians are genuinely busy, working long hours, driven by their patients' needs and line-ups in their waiting room. For so many, medical audit is a demand for time they do not have. There is neither a quick "in and out" to audit, nor any limit to its process. In accordance with Parkinson's Law, its demands expand to fill the time available.

The second perception is related to the first: *lack of reward.* No one ever gets anything useful from audits. As with so much research, audits just document the obvious or, after opening cavern after cavern of uncertainty, they themselves disappear into the black hole.

Medical audit is part of an *alien system:* it belongs to "them", and real clinicians are "us". Who "they" are we do not know — the government, administration, the College of Physicians and Surgeons, the Establishment. And "they" play political games with audits, with auditing practices they wish to expose, and with gathering data in order to do so.

Fourth, *confidentiality,* or the loss of it, poses a threat. Every batter fouls out sooner or later, but he does not need to have this news displayed on the big screen every time he goes up to bat. Medical audit teaches clinicians to cover themselves, to do whatever they must to avoid exposure. "Not seen as an educational process" is an understatement!

The fifth negative perception is the association of

medical audit with *discipline*. For physicians, audit and peer
review carry threats that QA does not pose to other staff.
The Manitoba chiefs mentioned that QA was seen as "a form
of policing"; there was "uncertainty about the process", and
it was "intimidating and discomforting to assess peers".
These speakers were giving voice to a deep-seated suspicion
of the purposes and methods of medical audit. They do not
wish to be audited themselves, and they don't wish to have
any part in auditing their colleagues. Auditing is a "them"
activity. If there is a line between medical discipline and
medical audit, many doctors do not know where it lies.

The point of discussing the widespread alienation from
medical audit here is to encourage physician leaders to take it
seriously and adopt strategies to combat both the fears and
the negative realities. There are no neat solutions: for *time,*
prescribe speed of audit, for example. Instead, audit must
supply needs that are felt in the doctors' professional culture.
Of course, leaders must declare war against unimportant,
politically motivated, inefficient, uncontrolled and esoteric
audits, all of which are occurring today somewhere in
Canada. But chiefs need more fundamental criteria to match.
Here are three:

- *Personal satisfaction.* At the end of the day, the MDs
  participating in the audit need to recognize that they
  derived something from it for themselves. Each may have
  his or her own locus of satisfaction — learning
  something, or solving an interesting clinical problem —
  but there needs to be an exchange which the participant
  values for the time spent.

- *Practice protection.* Participants should feel, as a result of
  the audit, that their own practice and that of their
  colleagues is made safer. This may occur because of a
  validation of present practice or as a result of heeding
  recommendations made by the audit team.

- *Peer support.* There are two ideas here: professional
  recognition, and the enjoyment of working on a team.
  If, as we maintain, QA is about good news and not bad

news, there should be in medical audit an opportunity to recognize good practice, either that of the individual or of the group (e.g., Emergency physicians, the Department of Paediatrics). Second, medical practice, particularly outside the hospital, tends to be individualistic and short of peer interaction and support. Participation on a medical audit team, if well led, can be gratifying at a social-professional level. And secondary gains are important to the continuance and support of this activity.

Five Practical Problems

In working with medical staff, I have recommended that however they manage it, doctors must overcome the five common inhibitors of medical QA. The "five Cs" are:

- *Confusion.* Dr. McGregor chided her audience of QA professionals with continually "moving the goal posts". Not only is QA a moving target (in that its demands have changed significantly in 1977, 1983, 1985 and 1991), but so is its language or jargon. Physicians today are unsure what it is they are meant to be doing in QA.

- *Competence.* Nothing creates more aversion than requirements to do what people do not feel competent to do. The fear of failure, of being shown up, is highly inhibiting. A minority of medical staff members have had the experience of carrying a medical audit through to completion.

- *Confidentiality.* There is a serious threat in some provinces that audit committee data and minutes are subject to discovery by the courts. This lack of legal privilege means that a physician may be compelled to testify against a colleague because of the former's participation in an audit committee.

- *Continuity.* Medical audit in many hospitals is like an annual in a flower garden: the fact that it bloomed luxuriantly last year seems unrelated to what will flower, or how brightly, in the same place this year. Medical staff leadership changes, and physician interest in QA burns out fast when it is pursued alone.

- *Co-ordination.* Even when everything else is taken care of and motivation, competence, participation and protection are all maximized, medical audit can grind to a halt because it is undermanaged. As soon as the committee rises, its members are engulfed by clinical demands. Rounds, full waiting rooms and telephones will drive out of the mind the conclusions, promises and questions with which the meeting concluded.

If these are the important inhibitors, then some prescriptions are in order. Five are proposed:

Prescriptions for Practice

Put Up Targets

The confusion of medical staff is real and legitimate, and it springs from two questions: What do we have to do? and, How do we do it? In Chapter 5 I attempted to provide a basic framework in which medical QA can be addressed. Someone — and it should be the MAC — needs to put numbers to my prescriptions and say how many meetings, how many audits, by which committees and departments. It makes sense for the MAC to set up its own medical staff QA Calendar. How to do it? requires a different type of answer.

Create a Source of Expertise

There is no reason to assume that physicians, because they have a medical degree, know how to carry through a medical audit. Many have some audit experience — but much of that may not be helpful. This comment is not intended to be snide. One of the great failings of medical audit is that it is pursued as if it were clinical research, with detailed, demanding large samples and over long duration. The major justification for having a medical QA committee is to centralize the staff's expertise in audit. Such committees should be made up of representatives from departments and committees with audit responsibility, and be dedicated to developing expertise and providing assistance to those who will be doing the audits. Such committees should find or create audit forms and pathways (such as those in Chapter 4), and learn other means of medical care appraisal, such as those detailed in the second half of this chapter. The other justification for having a staff QA committee is that it allows Tissue & Audit to continue its work of surveillance — of the operating suite, deaths, and significant risk indicators. QA committees are warned that staff physicians will want and expect them to carry out the audits themselves. Those who do so will lend support to the fiction that medical care appraisal is a specialist activity and not a general responsibility.

Make Rules for Documentation

Changing a government's ideas and getting legislation passed to protect QA proceedings from discovery is the slowest and least sure way to address the problem of confidentiality. Instead the staff, with whatever assistance it needs from hospital management and the hospital lawyer, should draw up some simple rules on the documentation of QA proceedings. These might include checklists of what should appear, such as:

- Date, time and place of meeting

- Those in attendance

- A generic description of the cases discussed by age, sex, diagnosis, previous history

- Their disposition

- Focus of interest in the discussion

- Recommended changes to or reinforcement of medical procedures, if any, and

- The officials responsible for their implementation.

Equally, such lists should identify what should *not* appear:

- Any identifiers of patient or clinician

- Any ascription to an audit participant of any judgement or recommendation he or she may have made

- Any suggestion of culpability. Misdiagnosis will occur, but is often justifiable in view of what was or could have been known.

Finally, detailed notes that may have been prepared for the information of the committee should either be prepared in numbered copies and all copies collected, or be put on overhead transparencies, both to be destroyed after the meeting. If lawyers get upset by this recommendation, they should be reminded that the primary data are in the health record and are secure; it is only the analysis of the data that has been discarded.

Stick to a Schedule

The continuity of patient care appraisal is bedeviled by two problems: audits never get started, and those that do, never end. The QA committee, as audit leader, needs to set and defend a model of audit that is "quick and dirty": important topic, limited focus, small sample, direct analysis, conclusions and recommendations for action; duration of audit, ± 90 days. If, on analysis, there appear to be no clear conclusions, the audit team can authorize expanding the sample size by another 50%, and then analyze the total sample. This kind of model should take care of those who demand 100 or 500 cases at the outset and then expand the scope of the study or number of variables that must be interrelated in the analysis. These studies seldom lead to changes in clinical practice — only to staff disaffection with the audit process.

The second prescription is that the time to organize the next audit is when the data collection has been completed for the previous one. The second audit team will be distinct from the first, as will its topic. In addition, audit teams start slowly, so QA committees should give them ample lead time as well as a designated facilitator or advisor from the committee. Only in this way will the MAC QA Calendar or schedule be met.

Present the Bill to Management

A third prescription is simpler and is given to the hospital's Chief Executive Officer: If you want a viable medical QA program with regular audits, you are going to have to provide dedicated support. That support should match the hospital's funding of administrative physicians, not in dollars, but FTE for FTE (full-time equivalent). Is the Chief remunerated on a half-time basis? Do chiefs of department receive an honorarium — in recompense for what time? Support to medical staff is of two kinds: management and technical. Management may come in the person of an administrative physician such as a VP or Director of Medical Affairs, or a hospital manager or assistant; the manager may be the hospital's QA co-ordinator or a senior secretary. In a smaller facility, an executive assistant could provide the continuity and co-ordination that physicians in practice invariably need. This person should keep and follow up on minutes, prepare agendas, carry communications between officers, departments and teams, all the while ensuring that physicians make the decisions and, with prompting, carry them through.

Technical help is provided almost exclusively by health records administrators (HRA), and their time dedicated to audit and committee work should be counted into the support budget. Although it may be hard to arrange, I recommend that each medical department have a designated HRA as its technical support for audit, utilization and indicator purposes. Certainly each audit team will have its health records staff member named at the beginning of the project.

This section of the chapter ends with the reminder that patient care appraisal is an activity in which *all* physicians (on a staff of 100-150 *active* members) will expect to participate once every two years, or more frequently.

6.2
Charting the Territory

Some audit topics choose themselves; most don't. Thus, the lack of a viable topic emerges as one of the first turn-offs in medical audit: "We couldn't find a topic that interested any of us enough." This is a fair comment in an unstructured environment. The need is to provide the structure in which topics can be chosen, rather than depend on crises or individual interests. To do this we must go back to the basics, those presented in Chapter 2:

> *Quality assurance is an information system that allows us to answer on a repeat basis two questions: How well are we doing our job? and, How do we know?*

"Our job" was defined for hospital departments in terms of principal functions. We answered the question, "How do we know?" by finding data from patients, audits, indicators and outside experts. We shall recommend the same answers to medical staff.

Principal Functions

Whether among a small unified or a departmentalized medical staff, principal functions define the clinical workload — what staff do most. A small staff can say, with little hesitation, that they run a twenty-four hour Emergency department, do obstetrics and general surgery; they provide care to a twenty-four bed Chronic Care unit, and their Family Medicine staff treat, in order, heart conditions, respiratory complaints, and digestive problems.

From this description may come the following principal function list:

1. Emergency & Evacuation

2. Obstetrics & Newborn

3. Surgery

4. Chronic Care

5. General Medicine

In consequence, that staff's task is to set up a system by means of which the effectiveness of the major aspects of its care are monitored, assessed, improved, and reported.

Even if the staff needing to identify principal functions is the Department of Medicine, the task is only one step more sophisticated. Most medical departments will need to go back to their Hospital Medical Records Institute (HMRI) data to validate the clinical priorities they have estimated from experience. In this step they will use the HMRI accreditation print-out which gives the previous year's leading diagnoses (off the discharge summaries) and most frequent procedures. The leading diagnoses will be expressed in case-mix groups (CMGs); departments will need to group these into their major clinical categories (MCCs), so as to arrive at their principal (clinical) functions.

Thus the Department of Medicine at one community hospital, on the basis of its total patient days, could have elected to use the following principal functions:

1. Cardiovascular conditions

2. Nervous system/CVAs

3. Respiratory complaints

4. Digestive problems

Because of the number of subspecialists on staff, that did not recommend itself. Instead, the department chose:

1. Assessment and diagnosis

2. Clinical management

3. Disposition and followup, including patient/family education, referrals, etc.

4. In-patient consults, out-patient clinics

The department of Paediatrics in the same hospital combined clinical definition with generic functions:

1. In-patient care, divided into four important components: Respiratory (1730 days), Digestive (1023 days), ENT (724 days), and Other (?)

2. Assessment and care of newborn

3. Paediatric emergency

4. Consults to family practice

5. Staff and family education

Performance Assessment

Once a department has arrived at its principal functions it is in a position to ask and answer the question: How well are we doing our job? In Chapter 4, I proposed that a department's performance be assessed from four viewpoints — those of the patient or client, the team (audit), its outcomes or indicators, and outside assessors or experts. While these methods or viewpoints are alternatives, I suggested that assurance would come best from the congruence of data from all four sources. Here we will touch briefly on patient data and expert data. Later in this chapter we shall consider the use of outcome indicators and professional assessment or audit.

As Others See Us: Patients

I have no special insight to offer here on this topic; Chapter 4 treated it in detail. But for physician readers, it is worth making three points: First, I was myself convinced by Kaplan and Ware [1] of the validity of data from patients. Second, communicating with patients is not just good care; it is also prudent care from a risk perspective.[2] Third, clinicians are joining with managers to insist that satisfying the customer is the hallmark of quality improvement.[3] For these reasons, and because getting insightful data from patients is relatively easy, physicians are advised to consult Chapter 4 for methods of hearing from them. They will remember that the task in QA is for clinicians to learn *enough* either to change their behaviour or to continue in it with confidence.

As Others See Us: The Experts

Hospitals, as we have seen, are subject to multiple inspections by regulatory and governmental agencies. There is a major difference between them and those who review medical practice: the latter are invited. Physicians will think first of the semiobligatory visitors — the accreditation surveyors, representatives of the Royal College or medical faculty who have to attest to the quality of clerkships, internships and residencies. Sometimes, too, the coroner suggests visiting the hospital, and is never denied an invitation.

What is recommended here is the invitation of clinical experts as a regular part of a medical staff's QA program. Wherever there is a community hospital *without* organized departments carrying on surgery, obstetrics and advanced medicine such as coronary care — and who can avoid that? — then there are two needs. These are, first, a means of handling peer review, when there are no peers on staff; and second, the review of the quality of general practice in the absence of clinical specialists. Every year, small community hospitals should arrange a clinical visit for each of their specialty functions. The physician-expert should do four things for the staff: first, inspect the clinical area and equipment; second, review twenty to thirty recent charts; third, conduct a CME session; and fourth, write a one-page report on the inspection, including recommendations, for the attention of the MAC and board of trustees. If the hospital's Chief of Staff wished the visitor to make a credentials note for a sole specialist, that would also be useful. Clinical experts can come from two sources. The best is university teaching hospitals or medical school faculties. Also acceptable are large hospital specialists who themselves are subject to qualified peer review.

Performance Indicators

Chapter 3 was devoted to the development and use of performance indicators. My support for them as a QA construct echoes that of the CHA, CMA, CNA *et al.,* and the CCHFA in Canada, the Joint Commission, and many health care agencies and regulatory bodies in the United States. Performance indicators are commended for use because they refer to (often clinical) outcomes, their data are easy to collect, and they target the attention of those who should take responsibility. There is, however, one prevailing problem in their use by medical staff. Indicators tend to focus entirely on the negative sequelae of care. For example, the 1992 JCAHO trauma indicators [4] are declared in the negative (9 of 12), in the positive (1), and without value judgement (2). All eight of the anaesthesia indicators are negative.[5] Similarly, Lang's "primary care practice indicators" [6] are set in the negative. The fact of the matter is that negative certainty is easier to state and observe than positive. Unfortunately, a surfeit of negative indicators can feed into physicians' learned aversion to QA and peer review. For this reason, staff should make every effort to find both positive indicators and categories that do not imply fault or blame. Length of stay, consultation rate, utilization rates, admission to service by category (elective, urgent, emergency) would be examples.

In the lists shown below, the Department of Medicine did well to avoid the monotony of negatives in the indicators it chose to monitor:

Medicine

1. Death rate for myocardial infarction (MI) compared to peer hospitals

2. Incidence of MI per population base

3. Admissions by category, by physician

4. Nosocomial infection rate for service

5. Utilization: Special Care Units (ICU, Telemetry, etc.)

6. Readmission rate:
   - 1 week, related
   - 1 month, related

7. Length of stay outliers, by service (excluding those awaiting placement)

Surgery

1. Deaths < 48 h

2. Complications

3. Errors in diagnosis

4. Cases with minimal pathology

5. Transfusion reactions

These surgeons "tell it like it is"!

In summary:

- The use of indicators allows a department to monitor the quality and — depending on the indicator — the efficiency and appropriateness of clinical performance.

- Indicators allow comparisons with the department's past performance and with that of similar departments.

- Indicators raise questions about performance that need to be investigated, either when the events occur or later, by audit.

- Indicators are not infallible measures but vital signs of what is happening, an efficient tool in a complex organization.

6.3
Medical Care
Appraisal

The following section describes fifteen methods for assessing medical care. I hope that physician readers derive some encouragement from this discussion. They may find it liberating to discover in care appraisal practical alternatives to the often tedious, scholastic and expensive criterion-referenced audit. A second source of encouragement is that five of the methods focus on improvement rather than on sterile measurement. Medical audit is much more than a "blame accounting" system.

In discovering these many strategies I am indebted to two texts in particular: *Quality Assurance in Hospitals: Strategies for Assessment and Implementation,*[7] edited by N.O. Graham, and *Medicare: A Strategy for Quality Assurance,*[8] by K.N. Lohr. Both are excellent sources of strategies. In presenting the variety of methods available to practitioners, I have chosen to group them according to their central purpose: case- or problem-finding ("Finding the Hot Spots"), care assessment ("Evaluation Methodologies"), or improvement ("Strategies for Improvement"). In doing this I run the risk of offending devotees of various methods who may claim that their chosen method is designed to achieve all three objectives. But we have faced this issue in respect of QA and will do so also with CQI. Strategies in health management may *intend* to do all things, but *tend* to do only one or two really well and exhibit weaknesses at other points. There is no one strategy that will allow us to monitor, assess, prevent risks, and improve efficiency and clinical outcome. Instead, the challenge to physicians and hospital quality managers is to apply the most appropriate strategy to the problem or need presented.

Finding the Hot Spots

Patient Surveys

Patients' evaluation of their care was discussed fully in Chapter 4 and earlier in this chapter. The point to be made here is that surveying patients is a way of casting a wide net to see what is there, to ascertain how satisfied patients are with the physician's delivery of care.

Occurrence Screening

Occurrence screening is one of the foremost systems of problem finding or risk identification. Under this system, every in-patient chart is screened every forty-eight hours for any of a limited number of specific and negative occurrences. The handling of the evidence and the event are described in Chapter 8. All that needs to be observed here is that occurrence screening is a most effective system of identifying adverse patient occurrences concurrently — often well in time to address their effects with the patient while still in the facility.

Staging

Both this and the next method of care appraisal are triggered by predictable outcomes. The reasoning for staging [9] is as follows: If a disease process can be described in recognizable stages, then the patient's arrival at a later or more deteriorative stage raises the question of that patient's clinical management during the preceding stage(s). This logic is being followed by hospitals that routinely review patient referrals to other hospitals and in-patient admission to ICU. It can also be used in family practice to review coronaries in postcoronary patients, or admission of known diabetics for management of a deteriorative condition, such as circulatory problems. Once again, this is a case-finding method, rather than one that prescribes methods of investigation or improvement.

Sentinel Health Events

Graham describes this method: "Sentinel health events, the other outcome-based approach, utilizes the occurrence of preventable disease, avoidable complications, and untimely deaths as warning signs of suboptimal care." [10] In an article [11] she includes to define this method, the authors present three lists of more than 100 preventable conditions. These conditions are subdivided into lists of lessening certainty of antecedent medical neglect: (a) clear-cut, immediate-use indexes, (b) limited-use indexes, and (c) categories demanding special study. Although these lists will be of most interest to public health authorities because of their heavy emphasis on preventable disease, the method is readily adaptable to hospitals if the sentinel events chosen are based on in-patient care — complaints, complications, patient incidents (e.g., falls), readmissions, deaths. Through skillful choice of different sentinel events, this method can help identify salient problems in family practice.

Evaluation Methodologies

There are seven methods of medical audit whose primary focus is the evaluation of the care provided. Three are very familiar to hospital physicians: individual case reviews, structured reviews, and the criterion-referenced audit. Two more are well known from experience: the HMRI care appraisal program (CAP) and, from the literature, the monitoring and evaluation process of the American Joint Commission. The remaining two methods — the tracer method and practice pattern analysis — will be new to many readers.

Individual Case Review

Highly familiar to physicians is the conduct of such individual case reviews as autopsies, investigation of special incidents (including patient complaints), and case conferences. Often these will be carried out by some authority — committee or medical officer — as hospital policy.

Structured Reviews

There are, in most hospitals, certain categories of medical intervention that are routinely subject to structured review: blood usage (particularly single-unit transfusions), operations on female reproductive organs with or without consults, operations that are screened for surgical necessity (e.g., appendectomies, tonsillectomies), and cases where there is *prima facie* conflict between preoperative and postoperative (tissue) diagnosis.

The Criterion-Referenced Audit

The criterion-referenced audit (CRA) was presented as one of three fundamental methods of assessing professional performance in Chapter 4 (pp. 76-81). That account included descriptions of the several steps in audit and supplied a planning protocol (pp. 84-87). A description of the second method — the focussed study — followed (pp. 81-83) in the same detail. The third method, the data-based audit, is described on page 174 as the Care Appraisal Programs of HMRI. Physician readers are advised to consult the earlier material cited or — where they can be found — friendly texts in the medical literature. Criterion-referenced audits are more than native common sense. They demand patience, imagination, and clarity of purpose.

In spite of many physicians' antipathy towards criterion-referenced audits (because of their detail, many steps, large sample sizes, and poor yield in terms of clinical insight), there is a place for these audits. They are the gold standard for medical audit, and if engaged in intelligently can be made to work for busy practitioners. Unfortunately, when their discipline is revered too highly, it can control the users rather than the converse. Appropriate control would mean limiting the scope of the audit (e.g., four to six key questions), the size of the sample, and the period of practice under review. The major distinction that needs to be made is between audit for the purposes of clinical review and assurance, and clinical research for the development of valid, generalizable clinical standards. QA is interested in the practicality of the first rather than the scholarship of the second. This is the choice that will justify smaller audits.

McMaster University has contributed scholarship and expertise to the practice of medical care appraisal. The audit map shown in Exhibit 6.1 is taken from the Chedoke-McMaster Hospitals' audit manual;[12] it follows closely that found in the OHA-OMA *Patient Care Appraisal Handbook,* to which its staff contributed.[13]

Exhibit 6.1
Steps in the Problem-Based Audit Process

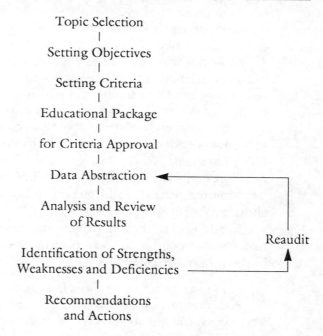

Topic Selection
|
Setting Objectives
|
Setting Criteria
|
Educational Package
|
for Criteria Approval
|
Data Abstraction ◄────────┐
| │
Analysis and Review   │
of Results   │
                    Reaudit
Identification of Strengths,
Weaknesses and Deficiencies ─────┘
|
Recommendations
and Actions

— Baynham, R. (1984). *Problem-Based Clinical Audit Handbook.* Hamilton, Ontario: Chedoke-McMaster Hospitals.

The Care Appraisal Programs (CAP) of HMRI

In the discussion of audit in Chapter 4, I referred to a data-based review. The HMRI CAP programs are the best-known Canadian model of review using a clinical data base. The mandatory abstracting of all in-patient charts for deposit in the HMRI data base means that data on a hospital's practice can be retrieved electronically in response to programmed instructions. A hospital wishing to engage in such a care appraisal program has two choices. Under CAP 1, its medical staff can determine which criteria it wishes to use in order to evaluate the care of a given group of patients. These criteria may require special data entry at time of abstracting, because no program can retrieve what has not been deposited. After the program has been run, the special data entry protocol can be terminated.

Most hospitals, particularly those with a small staff or one inexperienced in audit, will choose CAP 2, HMRI's second option. With the help of panels of clinical experts, HMRI has developed some twenty audit packages for such specific clinical conditions as cholecystectomy, Caesarean section, appendectomy, myocardial infarction, TURP, acute CVA, Emergency Room management of (non-ethanol) overdoses, psychotropic drug — lithium, management of the head-injured patient, and Emergency Room evaluation of abdominal pain.[14]

In addition to these care appraisal programs, HMRI issues routine reports on adverse patient occurrences found in the hospital's abstracts, such as:

> . . . *complication rates, adverse drug reactions, patient misadventures, anaphylactic shock, pulmonary embolism, complications of delivery, child maltreatment reactions, and sports injuries, etc.*[15]

HMRI advises that each hospital should have a mechanism to ensure that data on the above are reviewed on a continuing basis.

Monitoring and Evaluation Process

The literature contains many references to the ten-step monitoring and evaluation process of the Joint Commission in the United States.[16] This process depends on the development of performance indicators and prescribes how they can be used in the maintenance of professional standards. The ten steps given in Exhibit 6.2 may be more

Exhibit 6.2
The Ten-Step Monitoring and Evaluation Model of the Joint Commission

---

1. Assign responsibility for monitoring and evaluation activities

2. Delineate scope of care provided by the organization

3. Identify important aspects of care provided by the organization

4. Identify indicators (and appropriate clinical criteria) for monitoring important aspects of care

5. Establish thresholds (levels, patterns, trends) for indicators that trigger evaluation of care

6. Monitor important aspects of care by collecting and organizing data for each indicator

7. Evaluate care when thresholds are reached in order to identify either opportunities to improve care or problems

8. Take actions to improve care or to correct identified problems

9. Assess effectiveness of actions and document improvement in care

10. Communicate results of monitoring and evaluations process to relevant individuals, departments, or services and to the organization-wide quality assurance program

— Lohr, K.N. (1990). *Medicare: A Strategy for Quality Assurance* (vol. II). Washington, D.C.: National Academy Press, p. 164.

---

elaborate than necessary, but their logic is sound. Rather than carry out a succession of criterion-referenced audits, a medical staff is advised to identify by department or specialty the risk and leading indicators (to use the terminology of this text) of performance. As data are accumulated and plotted monthly (or procedure by procedure), their discrepancy should trigger investigation, assessment and remediation.

Performance indicators are commonly used by medical staffs, particularly in quality control, whose monitoring is often assigned to subcommittees of the MAC (see Exhibit 5.4, p. 134). The monitoring and evaluation process can also be extended to both departments and *descriptive* indicators. Whenever there are aspects of practice targetted for improvement — length of stay, appropriateness of test orders, surgical cancellations or trauma response — the use and stepped-up monitoring of descriptive indicators may be warranted. In continuous quality improvement (CQI) protocols, there is a phase labelled "holding the gains". The use and monitoring of performance indicators is tailor-made for that purpose.

Practice Pattern Analysis (PPA)

Recently the American Hospital Association developed a text, *Practice Pattern Analysis: A Tool for Continuous Improvement of Patient Care Quality.* [17] PPA seeks to review the characteristics of groups of doctors, such as whole departments or specialty teams, instead of measuring individual practice against guidelines or clinical yardsticks. PPA is described a "a method of aggregating data by practitioner, diagnosis, diagnosis-related group (DRG) or other defined category to show patterns of care and/or variations in treatment." [18] This audit method depends on five "basic elements for success":

1. Support, advocacy and active participation by physician leaders;

2. Clarification of the goals and uses of practice pattern analysis;

3. Careful management and communication of data;

4. Institutional support; and

5. Patience and perseverance.[19]

   The AHA text provides some dozen success stories from different U.S. facilities, from open-heart surgery to orthopaedics and obstetrics. PPA succeeds because it is data driven and pattern oriented rather than particular and regulatory. This newer method of medical care appraisal is highly compatible with CQI/TQM and appears to appeal to clinicians.

Strategies for Improvement

We come finally to a handful of strategies whose avowed intent is the improvement of practice. Some involve the gathering of data, but data are used either to find functioning problems that are in need of remediation or to monitor the success of the remedy applied.

Clinical Reminder Systems

The clinical reminder system [20] is an automated, on-screen, physician-developed system that gives the clinician immediate feedback — reminders of appropriate action — when he or she types in the patient's symptoms and diagnosis. These systems do not measure the quality of care, but they improve it by inhibiting common errors and proposing tested generic clinical pathways.

Criteria Mapping

Criteria mapping [21] is a method of clinical description that informs, in the first instance, those who develop the algorithm or map. The power of flow charting of any kind lies in its success in objectifying the process, so that it can be reviewed and discussed without threat or rancour. A criteria map allows clinicians to review the complexity of a patient care process, sometimes to simplify it and often to highlight the critical steps in the process. The steps identified can be reinforced by consensus of the specialists and made the focus of standard setting and audit.

Practice Guidelines

There are currently few aspects of medical quality that cause such division as the proposal of practice guidelines, parameters or protocols.[22] One group says they are essential and effective; another that they are a recipe for "cookbook medicine". I have found myself wanting to persuade those who want practice guidelines for regulatory purposes to ease up, to stop acting like police. Meanwhile, I wish the "cookbook medicine" protesters would understand that their clinical judgement is heavily required to answer how and to what extent the guidelines would fit *this* patient. But this is a doctor-doctor battle, and there are significant arguments on both sides, including the difficulty of getting clinical experts to agree on standards and guidelines.

Both sides may well be able to support practice pattern analysis (see above) because of its use of aggregated data, its neutrality and pragmatism. Sometimes it may be just the words and their emotional freight that get in the way. One medical staff that I worked with developed a practice of turning a clinical risk or problem into an algorithm, and circularizing the recommended clinical path to all members of staff. As well as keeping them up to date, these pathways were good risk prevention, and established a norm that clinicians could point to if their case went sour — the pathway became a defence. Hospitals and physicians might see that as an asset.

The Comprehensive Quality Assurance System (CQAS)

Also compatible with CQI is a clinical improvement model dating back to 1973: the comprehensive quality assurance system.[23] CQAS is a method of solving clinical problems by adopting standards set by a consensus of staff. Like some other methods, CQAS is not particularly interested in measuring practice except to ensure that its solutions are working. Even after twenty years, CQAS still sounds modern to CQI ears. Exhibit 6.3 lists some of its characteristics.

Exhibit 6.3

Comprehensive Quality Assurance System (CQAS)

1. Does *not* depend on: abstract, coding, chart format; computer, electronic data processing, *any* data base; style of practice (fee-for-service or prepaid) or disease orientation (missed diagnosis problem)

2. Primarily addresses problems

3. Based on improvement (evaluation built in)

4. Comprehensive
   A. Setting — ambulatory, hospital, long-term care, etc.
   B. Performance improvement of: physician, nurse, patient, ancillary services, etc.
   C. Timing — concurrent or retrospective

5. Addresses many (not all) kinds of problems
   A. Quality (process or outcome)
   B. Utilization (over or under)
   C. Medico-legal hazards

6. Economical operation

7. Short lead time to improvement

8. *Locally* determined standards or criteria

9. Minimizes practitioner (physician, nurse, etc.) time, expense.

— Rubin, L. and Kellogg, M.A. (1982). "The Comprehensive Quality Assurance System." In: Graham, N.O., ed., *Quality Assurance in Hospitals*. Rockville, MD: Aspen, pp. 199-219.

Health Accounting

The name of this system hides more than it informs. Health accounting is a quality improvement system that is directed towards clinical problems identified by an epidemiological (hence health accounting) review of patient outcomes. Improvement is accomplished by an iterative process:

> Definitive assessment —> Improvement action —>
> Outcome reassessment (and recycle to Step #1).

The developers of this method were John Williamson and his colleagues at Johns Hopkins University. While Dr. Williamson is still contributing to the development of quality management, he may have left this method far behind. The major article [24] describing this model is dated 1975.

Using Other People's Models

When I want information I hate it if people give me a shopping list. Such lists seldom demonstrate priorities, whether of importance or application. In spite of this, what I have given readers in this chapter is essentially an annotated shopping list. Without a medical degree or experience of these methods, I have done what the researcher must do: lay out the evidence without prejudice. Medical QA committees are encouraged to track down these methods one by one, over a period, and evaluate the usefulness of each for their facility.

The racing fraternity has a saying, "Horses for courses" — meaning that some horses are better suited to the terrain of a particular course than others. These are the likely winners. This analogy applies to models of care appraisal. A staff that rebels against practice guidelines may be very supportive of practice pattern analysis. Another staff, not persuaded of the necessity for the introspection of audit, may be more convinced after coming to terms with evidence of poor care discovered by patient surveys or occurrence screening. But all this presupposes that someone (the chief or chiefs) or some group (the QA or Tissue & Audit committee) take responsibility for plotting a strategy to involve staff in the habitual assessment and improvement of their clinical practice. Effective medical audit presupposes leadership.

6.4
Medical Care
Appraisal and CQI

But there are two more serious objections to the laundry list of methods for assessing medical care. Both have to do with continuous quality improvement, and their seriousness for the reader will depend on how involved his or her hospital and medical staff are in implementing CQI/TQM.

In treating QA, medical QA, utilization and risk management in separate chapters, this book is inadvertently misleading. Its arrangement suggests that each of these quality strategies can be pursued on its own, without reference to the others. This section suggests that medical quality can be pursued by physicians in isolation from the non-medical people and hospital systems that provide the essential context in which the physician plays a role, albeit a central one. If CQI teaches only one lesson, it is that quality of service depends not on the individual, but on the soundness of the service delivery *process,* in which many people play a part. It is reckoned that only fifteen per cent of error is attributable to causes not intrinsic to the process. Individual error may be an important factor within this fifteen per cent. "In this context," writes Lang, "the responsibility of the medical staff is to develop a collaborative problem-solving relationship with other professionals in the hospital." [25] While the medical staff may never lose the responsibility for the quality of care provided by physicians, its isolated measurement, discussion and attempts at remediation will, under CQI, become a thing of the past. Instead, physicians will increasingly find themselves, on the nomination of their department or the MAC, serving on multidisciplinary quality improvement teams, in order to improve the clinical processes essential to high-quality care.

The second possible quarrel with the recital of methods is the author's failure to distinguish between methods that are of the present *and future* from those that are clearly of the past. Medical care appraisal has tended to be static, frozen sections of care, and its consideration diagnostic, individual and prescriptive. Physician proponents of CQI look for step-wise improvement, the regular meeting of improving standards, and shared pleasure in making things happen. A CQI medical staff will make frequent use of performance indicators, may be interested in methodologies to "find the hot spots", may find little use for the evaluation methodologies except for Practice Pattern Analysis, but will use the strategies for improvement either on their own or, more frequently, within the context of clinical CQI projects.

Addendum:
Topics of Medical Audit, Ontario 1989-1991

Early in 1991 the Ontario Hospital Association's Department of Medical Staff Affairs surveyed member hospitals as to their medical staff organization and audit activities. The findings of this important inquiry have been documented in a monograph published by the Association [26] and a subsequent article in the medical literature.[27] Medical staffs frequently comment on the difficulty of finding good audit topics. Accordingly, and with the assistance of the authors of the OHA study, I have reproduced, by specialty, lists of topics that medical staffs and organized departments claim to have carried out in the two years prior to survey (see Exhibit 6.3). As lists of important, good or common topics, they are patently incomplete. However, they should prime the pump for those undertaking audit responsibility for the first time.

Exhibit 6.4
Topics of Medical Audits Carried Out in Hospitals in Ontario1989-1991, by Specialty

Internal Medicine
- TPN Administration
- Medical Consultations
- Effectiveness of Streptokinase
- Myocardial Infarction
- Diabetes Mellitus Management
- Management of Hypertension
- Use of NSAIDS
- Administration of Pulmonary Function Tests
- Emergency Transfers
- Treatment of Urinary Tract Infection
- Adverse Drug Reactions
- Microbiology Specimen Audit

Surgery
- Anaesthesia Chart Audit
- Amputations
- Deaths within 48 h Post-op
- Admission After Out-patient Surgery
- Cardiac Surgery Waiting List
- Results of Open-Heart Surgery
- Pulmonary Embolism
- Cholecystectomy
- Complications Audit

Obstetrics and Gynaecology

Caesarean Section Rates

Primary C-Sections — Complications

Vaginal Births After C-Sections

Induction of Labour

Pelvic Inflammatory Disease

Culdoscopy Service

Out-patient Gynaecology Procedure

Psychiatry

Psychotropic Drug Therapy

Antiparkinson Medication Reaudit ECT

Adequacy of Discharge Planning

Postsuicide — Chart Audit

Poly-Pharmacy Audit

Emergency

Waiting Time in ER

Return to ER within 48 h

Interpretation of X-rays in ER

Management of:
- Ankle injuries, knee injuries
- Cardiac arrest
- Head Injuries — Emergency/OR
- Abdominal Pain
- Physician Documentation in ER
- Pharyngitis

Family Practice

Wheezing/Asthma

Diabetes

Pain Control in Terminally Ill

In-patient Cardiac Fatalities

Annual Assessments/Health Reviews

Prescribing Practices in the Elderly

Respite Bed Program

Continuous Bladder Irrigation

Ophthalmology
- Cataract
- Cataract Surgery
- Efficiency of Nd-Yag Laser Iridotomy
- Graft Rejection and Graft Failure

Other Specialities

Paediatrics
- Newborn Transfers to Larger Centres
- Circumcisions
- Neonatal Jaundice Management

Anaesthesia
- Complications of General Anaesthesia

Urology
- Continuous Catheter Drainage
- Urological Investigations in Women with Recurrent GU Tract Infections

Laboratories
- Use of Endococcal Bacterium Lab Results
- Microbiology Specimen Audit
- Colonoscopy
- X-ray Reports Compared to Autopsy Findings

ENT
- Sinusitis
- Complications of Tonsillectomy

References

1. Kaplan, S.H. and Ware, J.E. (1989). "The Patient's Role in Health Care and Quality Assessment." Chapter 2 in: Goldfield, N. and Nash, D.B., eds., *Providing Quality Care: The Challenge to Clinicians*. Philadelphia: American College of Physicians, pp. 25-68.
2. Cunningham, L. (1991). *The Quality Connection in Health Care*. San Francisco: Jossey-Bass, pp. 47n, pp. 98-99.
3. Berwick, D.M. (1989). Continuous improvement as an ideal in health care. *New England Journal of Medicine 320* (1 [5 Jan.]):55. See also: Laffel, G. and Blumenthal, D. (1989). The case for using industrial-quality management science in health care organizations. *Journal of the American Medical Association (JAMA) 262*(20 [24 Nov.]):2869-2870.
4. Joint Commission on Accreditation of Healthcare Organizations (1992). *Accreditation Manual for Hospitals*. Oakbrook Terrace, IL: JCAHO, pp. 230-231.
5. *Ibid.,* p. 22.
6. Lang, D.A. (1991). *Medical Staff Peer Review*. Chicago: AHA, p. 62.
7. Graham, N.O., ed. (1982). *Quality Assurance in Hospitals*. Rockville, MD: Aspen.
8. Lohr, K.N. (1990). *Medicare: A Strategy for Quality Assurance*. Washington, D.C.: National Academy.
9. Gonnella, J.S., Louis, D.Z., and McCord, J.J. (1976). The staging concept — An approach to the assessment of outcome of ambulatory care. *Medical Care 14*:13-21. Reprinted in: Graham, *op. cit.,* pp. 239-249.
10. Graham, *op. cit.,* p. 144.
11. Rutstein, D.D. *et al.* (1976). Measuring the quality of medical care: A clinical method. Originally published in: *New England Journal of Medicine 294*(11 [11 March]):582-588. Reprinted in: Graham, *ibid.*
12. Baynham, R. (1984). *Problem-Based Clinical Audit Handbook*. Hamilton, Ont.: Chedoke-McMaster Hospitals, p. 2.
13. Ontario Hospital Association/Ontario Medical Association (1982). *Patient Care Appraisal Handbook*. Toronto: OHA, p. 24.
14. These lists of conditions and occurrences are taken from an untitled, undated description of HMRI services issued 1989, 1990.

15. *Ibid.*
16. Joint Commission on Accreditation of Healthcare Organizations (1986). Monitoring and evaluation of the quality and appropriateness of care: A hospital example. *Quality Review Bulletin (QRB) 12*(9 [Sept.]):327-328.
17. American Hospital Association (1991). *Practice Pattern Analysis: A Tool for Continuous Improvement of Patient Care Quality.* Chicago: AHA.
18. *Ibid.*, p. 7.
19. *Ibid.*, pp. 16-19.
20. Donaldson, M.S. and Lohr, K.N. (1990). "A Quality Assurance Sampler: Practice Guidelines and Algorithms." In: Lohr, *op. cit.*, vol. II, pp. 201-206.
21. Greenfield, S., Lewis, C.E., Kaplan, S.H., and Davidson, M.B. (1975). Peer review by criteria mapping: Criteria for diabetes mellitus. *Annals of Internal Medicine 83*:761-770; see also: Black, M., Van Berkel, C., Green, E., Everett, I., and Krilyk, J. (1989). Criteria map: Potential for skin breakdown — A quality assurance tool for use in any setting. *QRB(Nov.)*:340-346.
22. Donaldson & Lohr, *op. cit.* (see Note 20); also, College of Physicians and Surgeons of Ontario (1990). *Proceedings of Independent Health Facilities Workshop.* Toronto, Ont., 29-30 November 1990.
23. Rubin, L. and Kellogg, M.A. (1982). "The Comprehensive Quality Assurance System." In: Graham, *op. cit.*, pp. 199-219.
24. Williamson, J.W., Aronovitch, S. *et al.* (1975). Health accounting: An outcome-based system of quality assurance. *Academy of Medicine 51*(6):727-738.
25. Lang, D.A. Personal communication, 25 August 1992.
26. Barrable, B. and Dawson, H. (1991). *Medical Staff Organization and Quality Assurance.* Toronto: OHA.
27. Barrable, B. (1992). A survey of medical quality assurance programs in Ontario hospitals. *Can. Med. Assoc. J. 146*(2 [15 Jan. 15]):153-160.

7

Utilization Review and Management

Utilization review (UR) — or, to give it its Canadian name, utilization review and management (URM) — comprises two complementary systems: a *data system* which provides an analysis of the use of important hospital resources, principally in-patient accommodation, intensive care beds and operating room bookings, and a political or *management system* through which the benefits of these and other resources are maximized. URM allows management and medical staff to answer such basic questions as:

- What is the hospital's clinical profile, in terms of the volume and variety of patient services provided?

- What proportion of patients from its community is the hospital treating?

- How appropriate is the use of hospital beds, in comparison with their use by other facilities in the province or the country?

- Are there procedures being carried out that might be handled by less expensive means?

- Is the hospital treating those most in need of care?

- Are patients being discharged earlier than their condition warrants?

Underlying URM are two presumptions. First, hospital and health care resources are finite and insufficient to meet all the demands that patients and physicians might make of them. If patients are not to be put at risk, resources must be allocated with extreme prudence, so that care is available to those in need. Second, there is general recognition that the least care is usually the best care. Hospitals are not benign environments; adverse patient occurrences are surprisingly frequent. In the United States the estimate is that one patient in five (20%) is likely to have an adverse patient occurrence in the course of a ten-day stay. (This phenomenon is discussed more fully in Chapter 8, "Managing Risk in the Department".) There are many examples in the clinical literature showing a concurrence of high volume, good outcome, and short stay.

This chapter will look at four aspects of URM: first, the use of data systems; second, the operation of the physician-driven management system; third, the management of clinical resources that are not available for review through the in-patient record; and fourth, outcomes management.

7.1
Use of Data
Systems

Hospital Medical Records Institute

In most provinces all hospitals are required to code and abstract information (often on disk) on all patients, and forward it to the Hospital Medical Records Institute (HMRI). This rich, enormous and current data base allows HMRI to perform a range of analyses on a hospital's clinical experience in comparison with itself, to the level of the individual physician, and in comparison with matched cases.

(Matched cases are cases in the data base of similar diagnosis without significant co-morbid conditions.)

Hospital utilization is anchored to the concept of length of stay (LOS) — how long individual patients or groups of patients remain in the hospital. HMRI reports[1] can show a hospital its average LOS

- for total acute beds

- for total long-term beds

- by case-mix group (CMG)

- by procedure

and it will show these in comparison with the data base mean for matched cases. Columns in the same table will translate these comparisons with the mean into days potentially lost per case (if the facility's performance is greater than the mean LOS) or saved (if less than the LOS of the matched-case mean).

Other reports show the hospital's performance from the perspective of the day of admission; for example, Sunday and Monday admissions tend to have a lower LOS than patients admitted on Thursday and Friday. Similarly, completion of a surgical procedure within twenty-four hours of admission translates into lower lengths of stay.

But length of stay can also be too short. Physicians are encouraged to question one- and two-day in-patient stays. Were the admissions necessary? Was the procedure undertaken one that could just as well have been performed on an out-patient or day-surgery basis? There are published lists of "Possible Outpatient Surgical Procedures" and "Possible Day-Medicine Programs".[2]

Professional judgements will also be influenced by the route of admission. A Utilization committee is likely to view a two-day stay for an elective procedure that is on the possible out-patient list quite differently from the same procedure with the same LOS, when the patient was admitted through the Emergency department. For that reason the route of admission — emergency, urgent, or elective — is also listed with LOS data. This breakdown allows the hospital to maintain surveillance over emergency admissions, the traditional "back door" into the hospital for impatient physicians.

Utilization committees, whose mandate and composition are described below, need also to take cognizance of both early readmissions and admissions following day surgery. Both could raise questions of clinical judgement in that the LOS allowed in one case or planned for in another was not appropriate to the patient's condition. Both readmission within forty-eight hours of discharge and admission following day surgery are important *outcome indicators*. Their importance will be enhanced in the 1990s as Canada's health system continues to contract.

All of the HMRI data that are available to the hospital on its clinical performance are also available by physician, identified by ID number. Thus, doctors can examine their practice profile in comparison with those of their hospital peers and data base peers. Though these data are confidential, individual physicians and their hospitals can have access to them.

Ministry of Health Data

Hospitals would like to know that they are treating those most in need, and caring for them when necessary in the order of their need. Unfortunately, the data that are readily available to them do not answer these questions directly. Instead, through utilization management they can attempt to ensure that there is strong clinical justification for each in-patient day, OR booking, and ICU admission. They can also review information from their provincial Ministry of Health as to the domicile of their patients. Ministries of health routinely analyze the domicile (by postal code) of the admissions to hospital, so that a city hospital, for example, can ascertain how many of its patients come from the city and its adjacent counties, or farther afield. While a hospital's profile is not accessible to its neighbours, all profiles are available to District Health Councils and their consultants, for planning purposes. Increasingly, hospitals are going to wish to ensure that they are fulfilling their "social contract" in treating patients from their community and catchment area, within the limits of their clinical competence. On the other hand, they will wish to ensure that their resources are not being unfairly burdened because neighbouring facilities are failing to carry their weight. Bed closures to cut costs may profit hospital A, but if the result is merely the shifting of its costs, hospitals B and C both have a right to bring the matter to the attention of hospital A and those involved in regional planning.

7.2
Utilization
Management

The key political insight in utilization is that resources will best be managed by those whose livelihood depends on using them. Thus, the basic rule is that hospital utilization is a physician-driven system of reviewing the efficiency with which scarce clinical resources are employed, and instituting and maintaining strategies to improve their day-to-day management. The *Guide to Hospital Utilization Review and Management* carries a more detailed definition:

> *Utilization management is a proactive, joint medical-staff/management process in which a hospital continually works towards maintaining and improving the quality of care through the effective use of resources. It is a commitment not only to review the hospital's utilization patterns but also to take action on any areas of inappropriate utilization.*[3]

This section reviews the organization of URM in a facility, and the terms of reference of a Utilization Management committee.

The Organization of URM

There are four ingredients to an effective structure for the hospital URM program. First, the board of trustees needs to assume responsibility for ensuring the effective management of the hospital's clinical — and operational — resources. This role is clearly demonstrated in the accreditation *Standards*.[4] In fact, since 1985 URM has been stipulated as a board responsibility. The locus of responsibility is important for two reasons: first, URM is linked with the hospital's responsibility to its community. Second, as long as the board takes ownership of URM it will not be allowed to deteriorate into a dogfight between the resource users (i.e., physicians) and the bill payors (hospital management).

The second constituency in the URM team is the primary stakeholders, the physicians themselves. Whatever URM calls for, doctors must implement it for and with other doctors. This means representation for all those doctors whose calls, blocks and space are to be constrained. All organized medical departments need to have a representative at the table.

Hospital management needs to be at the table too, in three capacities:

- *Honest broker.* Management does not have a stake in which service has which beds.

- *Essential link with line departments.* URM decisions that bind physicians also affect diagnostic and treatment departments, which need to get into step with changes agreed upon at this level.

- *Administrator of the URM program.* While physicians may make the decisions, management has a stake in seeing the process work.

Hospital management will provide space, secretarial support, health records and other backing — including coaching to the physician chair — in order to make the program work. Management should be represented by the CEO, the senior nurse executive, and perhaps the chief financial officer, in addition to representatives from Admitting, the Operating Suite, Discharge Planning, and probably the Emergency department.

The fourth ingredient is the technical input to the committee and the process. Health records time and competence are two essentials. Equally important, there must be strong representation from the MAC's Tissue & Audit committee, which shares with Utilization a similar relationship with physicians, that of peer surveillance. It is highly appropriate to have physician representation from Laboratories and Radiology.

Terms of Reference

The terms of reference for a hospital's UR committee given in Exhibit 7.1 are taken from the 1988 OHA/OMA *Guide.* It is fuller in its text than the terms of reference given in the 1990 OHA/OMA *Prototype Hospital Bylaws.*[5] For some reason, its third item is not repeated in the later version. Item 3 says, in essence, that what is sauce for the goose is sauce for the gander — which sounds eminently fair. Why should utilization be a stick to beat only doctors with? The *Guide* describes, in separate chapters, various activities the committee should undertake in pursuance of its principal duties, e.g., reviewing:

- occupancy and length of stay
- admissions and readmissions
- consultations
- discharge procedures
- diagnostic and therapeutic services.[6]

Exhibit 7.1
UR Committee Terms of Reference

1. To review utilization patterns in the hospital to determine whether overall community needs are being met, and to identify where improvements in utilization patterns could be achieved.

2. To monitor regularly overall trends in admissions, length of stay and day program volumes, and provide appropriate information to Department Chiefs and Division Heads.

3. To review the utilization and efficiency of all hospital diagnostic, therapeutic and support services that affect the ability of the hospital to make effective use of its beds and other programs.

4. To ensure that department chiefs are educated about utilization review issues and methods and about their responsibility for reporting regularly to their departments on utilization trends.

5. To report findings and make recommendations on the above three areas to the MAC and administration on a monthly basis.

6. To receive and evaluate reports from medical staff departments on their monitoring of day-to-day utilization of beds.

7. To monitor response to those committee recommendations which are approved by the MAC and administration, and to report back on progress achieved.

8. To report annually to the full medical staff on the committee's activities.

9. To comment on the resource implications of proposed additional positions on the medical staff.

10. To perform such other duties as may be requested from time to time by the MAC.

— Adapted from: Ontario Hospital Association/Ontario Medical Association/Ontario Ministry of Health/Hospital Medical Records Institute (1988). *Guide for Hospital Utilization Review and Management in Ontario.* Toronto: OHA, p. 9.

The years that have passed since the publication of the *Guide* in 1988 have served only to underscore the importance of all these activities. In particular, the role of the utilization management committee in impact analysis (Exhibit 7.1, item 8) has been enhanced by time. In 1991, the OHA, OMA and HMRI published their *Guidelines for Medical Manpower Planning and Impact Analysis in Hospitals.* One paragraph in the executive summary reads:

> *Impact analysis and utilization review are distinct, but related, exercises. Impact analysis is a prediction of future utilization, whereas utilization review measures actual resource use in retrospect. Hospitals may find it useful to have the utilization review committee co-ordinate impact analysis activities in order to benefit from their expertise in data measurement.*[7]

7.3
Strategies in Managing Length of Stay

One of the first things that impresses the student of utilization management is that systems that succeed are complex rather than simple. Feferman and Cornell wrote a special article for the *CMA Journal* entitled, "How We Solved the Overcrowding Problem in Our Emergency Department." Their answer was:

- Establishment of a ten-bed Geriatrics Unit

- Reallocation of ten beds from Surgery to Medicine

- Establishment of a Short-Stay Unit and an Ambulatory Procedures Unit

- Inauguration of a physician-managed admission system (PMAS).[8]

Similarly, when the Greater Victoria Hospital Society (GVHS) took steps to address its utilization problems, its major departure was the introduction of severity of illness (S/I) and intensity of service (I/S) criteria for monitoring the appropriateness of admission, care and discharge. But other initiatives contributed to GVHS' success, including "same-day surgery, home care, improved liaison with community agencies, and the mobilization of a quick-response team for frail elderly in the community."[9]

Belleville General Hospital's URM program focussed on the publication of an expected date of discharge (EDD) on every in-patient chart at the time of admission.[10] However, the monitoring of emergency-admission and long-stay (> 30 days) patients was begun by the Utilization Review committee, and Discharge Planning was encouraged to seek out alternative placement strategies in the community.

From these and other accounts it appears that "success" in URM probably depends on at least six essentials: physician ownership, good data, published expectations, the employment of alternatives, a team approach, and support by management and the board.

Physician Ownership

In a1987 article Langelle tells how a medium-sized (135 + 50 bed) hospital complex in rural Alberta successfully addressed three chronic problems: high length of stay (8-9 days), long waiting lists for Medicine and Surgery, and the resulting continuous friction between physicians and between the medical staff and the hospital. A Utilization committee initiated a number of experimental systems over a four-year period before finding the key to the door:

> *Finally the medical staff proposed a by-physician bed allocation system. The medical staff argued that if they were to be held responsible for bed utilization as a group or as individuals then they should have the corresponding author-ity to manage the beds in a non-competitive manner.*[11]

And so they did. The medical staff allocated to each physician in accordance with his or her clinical privileges a maximum number of beds on each service. Where physicians had more claims than the beds available, some allocations were shared. Any physician wishing to exceed his or her allocation had to "borrow" a bed from another MD. Beds in ICU, Obstetrics, and Day Surgery were unallocated. In addition, a set number of beds on each service was reserved for emergency admissions. These beds were to be cleared within twenty-four hours, so that emergency beds were always available.

Today's readers may conclude that this system would never work in their hospital, but it succeeded in Wetaskiwin dramatically and over a sustained period. The hospital's mean LOS declined from an average of 8.4 days (1977-80) to a low of 5.8 days (1984-85); occupancy (84% average) fluctuated around 76% in the four years (1981-85) following introduction of the system, and the hospital's admissions increased from a mean of 4877 to 6323 patients in 1984-85. Langelle does not give figures for waiting lists or delays in treatment, but indicates that they were, at the time of writing, a thing of the past. As to the constant friction over bed availability, he concludes: "These changes have greatly improved the working relationship between physicians as well as with hospital staff."[12] The article's title identifies the solution: "Wetaskiwin Physicians Manage Bed Allocations."

In spite of the risk of repeating principles enunciated earlier, physicians' role in URM must be stressed, first as stakeholders. Medical staff have a direct interest in seeing the hospital's resource allocation system work, both for themselves (as entrepreneurs) and for their patients (with the MD as advocate). Second, physician leadership in such a sensitive area is the only leadership with any credibility. Harrison and Roger use the term "champions" to denote physicians who went out on their own in support of GVHS' utilization measures. Third, to the extent that the medical staff is a self-regulating society, its official leaders must be seen to advocate and implement the systems chosen. Fourth, clinicians who are sensitive to patient data need to maintain the client perspective within the body managing the utilization program.

Physicians who undertake leadership in utilization management seem to be transformed by the problem, discovering a commitment to the process as it unfolds. For them utilization means quality of care, improved accessibility, and increased patient satisfaction. There is also the recognition of interdependence, the reliance of physicians on each other and of medical staff on Nursing and other clinical departments, in bringing about necessary change.

Good Data

There is nothing that influences physicians like accurate and timely data. The Greater Victoria Hospital Society was prepared to bring in and adapt a fairly complicated American clinical assessment system. Its medical staff accepted and used the data. Scarborough General provided a dedicated personal computer so that each service's physician monitor could have up-to-the-minute information on the bed situation throughout the hospital. Belleville General's UR committee wanted HMRI's average length of stay (ALOS) data to be available to clinicians from the time of each patient's admission. The patient's ALOS was called, after conversion to the calendar, the "expected date of discharge" (EDD).

After the implementation of the EDD system, lengths of stay, by case-mix group (CMG), were compared with those of one year earlier.

> [Of 82 CMGs] 57 (70%) showed a decreased average length of stay (ALOS). Furthermore, during the first quarter of 1988-89, 44 (54%) of the 82 CMGs had an ALOS less than or equal to that calculated by HMRI. This figure improved to 60 (73%) [one year later].[13]

This "success story", as the article is titled, illustrates this aspect of physician behaviour; physicians are influenced by data. In his book on physician peer review, Lang gives an example of the appendectomy performance of two surgeons,[14] and quotes a prostatectomy study in which there was a comparison between the fastest surgeon (mean time, 25 min) and the slowest (100 min). Patients of the latter had more postoperative complications and a slower and more costly recovery. Lang continues:

> *Identification of these kinds of differences serves a variety of valuable functions. It has been shown repeatedly that physicians will respond to clinically valid information with self-correction. . . . The department chair can motivate individual physician improvement by sharing clinically specific performance information in a confidential setting. This approach is more likely to modify physician behaviour in a positive way than one that emphasizes restriction or limitation.*[15]

Published Expectations

Scarborough General Hospital reported the following in its newsletter:

> *The Department of Obstetrics/Gynaecology set target lengths of stay for normal deliveries (3 days) and Caesarean sections (5 days). Patients are informed of these targets before and during their admission, and achievement of the targets is monitored on a regular basis.*[16]

Published expectations are there for all to see! Average length of stay or EDDs are easiest to calculate and publish, but are the least flexible. The use of clinical measures such as MedisGroup indices or APACHE — two proprietary systems that score the acuity of the patient's condition — allows a hospital to monitor in-patient activity on a concurrent basis. This is done most frequently in respect of bed occupancy in

Intensive Care Units. Some tertiary-care hospitals have adopted the expectation that each in-patient day be justified by evidence of active care: postsurgical recovery, wound care, therapy including rehabilitation, invasive and other diagnostic procedures. They introduced chart monitoring systems to ensure that patients were under active care, and regularly question attending physicians whose patient management seems less active.

Less draconian are utilization and quality systems that depend on *case management* and *critical paths*. Case management is the co-ordination by one health care professional, usually a nurse, of all care provided to one patient. Case management is better known as a mental health strategy, often in community care, rather than a system for managing acute in-patients. Most of its development and literature comes from the New England Medical Centre Hospitals in Boston, where it was an outgrowth of many years of primary nursing (i.e., a designated RN assumes responsibility for each patient for the duration of his or her admission). The significant difference between case management and primary nursing is that while the patient's care is individually managed, it is managed in accordance with a critical path developed "for designated patients. . . admitted to a formally prepared group practice composed of an attending physician and a specific group of staff nurses from each of the units and clinics likely to receive these patients."[17] The critical path prescribes what episodes of care will occur on each day of the expected stay, including ICU, consults, tests, activity, treatments, diet, discharge planning, and teaching.[18] This system claims notable success in the treatment of a variety of patient conditions — ischemic stroke, adult leukaemia, and aortic aneurysm repair patients — with significant decreases in ALOS, intensive care days, and infection rates, as well as increased patient satisfaction and quality of life.

The Search for Alternatives

Scarborough General's physician-managed admission system was only one of fourteen steps taken by the hospital to address its bed management problems.[19] Band-aid solutions to Scarborough's overcrowded Emergency department could have meant more money, more space, more frequent closures to ambulance traffic and, of course, increased criticism of a larger number of targets. What was interesting about that hospital's response was that — if Feferman and Cornell[20] are to be believed — nothing particular was done about the Emergency department site or staff. Its problems were ameliorated when its root causes were addressed. Because poor utilization is the result of multiple malfunctions, it defies simple or unidimensional solution. Effective utilization is not a "quick fix".

All the Players, All the Time

Hospitals are complicated systems. Good utilization depends on everything coming together in the right order at the right time. For a single operation the bed, the preadmission diagnostic reports, the anaesthetist's visit, consent, blood, and OR time are just some of the necessary ingredients. To date, the major clinical impact of continuous quality improvement (CQI) has been in the improvement of patient systems. Hassen provides examples from the Operating Room, Emergency department and Obstetrics.[21] In the same journal, Schurman gives two examples of quality improvement team successes:

- Total hip replacement: 21% reduction in resources;

- Cholecystectomy: 23% reduction in resources. . . .[22]

The most important resource is staff time — paid hours.

Although so much of the responsibility for utilization management falls on physicians' shoulders, their best efforts can be nullified by poor systems or lack of co-operation. Key to URM is Nursing, Discharge Planning, data from Health Records, timely and accurate reports from Diagnostic Services — and the list goes on. URM is neither individual nor heroic. It demands communication, teamwork and a shared concern to make things happen better for the patient.

Last is the essential role of the board and senior management. There is every temptation for the board, having endorsed the URM policy, to walk away, saying, "It's up to you guys now." And of course, it is. But the board's continued interest in the results of the URM program is important to all participants. The board expresses a social, not just a finanacial, concern. It keeps the team playing the ball and not each other.

While management continues to preach the responsibility of clinicians for utilization management, it will provide all support necessary — including the CEO's presence at the table — to ensure that the system works.

7.4
Utilization Management in Diagnostic and Ancillary Services

URM is less developed in non-physician services and in physician-led diagnostic services. There are four probable reasons for this. First, the most expensive decisions — to admit, to test, to operate and to discharge — are made by individual physicians, and thus become the target for URM. Second, Dr. A's use of a bed or an operating room means that Dr. B cannot use the same space for her patients; utilization management is a self-protective program. Third,

URM can use similar rules and generic strategies in doctor services which it cannot duplicate for Radiology, Pharmacy, and Physiotherapy, for example. Fourth, and possibly most important, the critical decision in URM — that to test or treat — has already been made before the patient reaches the department.

With these provisos, three general directions can be advised to address appropriateness, efficiency, and overload. It is worth including a note on the handling of waiting lists, before mentioning one service-specific strategy.

Improving Appropriateness

If the decision to test or treat has already been taken, how can the affected department influence the appropriateness of the service that has been ordered? In two ways. If, on examination of the patient, the treating professional questions the usefulness of the therapy ordered, he or she should take a leaf from the pharmacist's book and recommend a substitution. Pharmacists routinely assess the appropriateness of the drug, dose, or route ordered, and are used to discussing alternatives with the ordering physician. If the substitution is clinically an improvement, or a behavioural strategy likely to be more effective, physicians will often concur.

The other avenue is post-treatment feedback. The treating professional's intent is to increase the appropriateness and perhaps timeliness of the physician's referral. Having done what was ordered, the former should take the opportunity to inform the physician how he or she might better serve that patient in the future. In this connection, I remember sitting in on a MAC executive meeting at a teaching hospital at which the chief of Laboratories was asking for steps to reduce the percentage of lab tests ordered *stat*. Apparently, every few years it was necessary to address the inevitable escalation in perceived urgency. *Stat* tests lowered the efficiency of the department, since they could

not be batched along with others and delayed the
performance of routine tests. The medical executive
understood the point well and authorized an approach to all
chiefs of department, who would take responsibility for
discussing inappropriate *stats* with members of their
department, residents and interns.

Increasing Efficiency

For the foreseeable future, Canadian hospitals will need to
place a premium on moving people through the system
more efficiently. Professional positions may be lost for
budgetary reasons, but the same volume of patients will
continue to present at the front door. CQI will probably help
the efficiency of service delivery, but departments — alone
and in discussion with others — are still going to have to
come up with better ways of managing workload. This may
include referral hospitals' accepting the validity of tests and
radiographs done by the referring facility. It will certainly
include the intent to make every treatment count to the
fullest, so as to limit the number and duration of returns to
therapy. It will probably mean fewer but more vital team
conferences.

Coping with Overload

There are two ways of coping with overload. One is to refuse
to compromise standards and offer treatment only to those
who can be accommodated within the resources available.
The other is to search for a variety of treatment modalities,
try them, test their efficiency and effectiveness, and use as
many as can offer specific benefits to particular clients in
particular situations. Two suggestions may help:

- The dominant pattern of treatment today is still 1:1 —
  one patient to one professional. Can the strengths of
  group support not be used to encourage the client and

assist the professional? Weight loss groups, diabetic education, group therapy, new mothers and postcoronary groups are obvious examples of areas where this strategy is already working.

- Another kind of group support is *family.* The patient and family may be "actively engaged as members of the health care team and *given specific responsibilities and control.*"[23] Family members can become the adjuvants of choice in rehabilitation, if they can be taught to respect the patient's need to make choices.

Handling Waiting Lists

There are few questions asked more frequently by professionals serving out-patient populations than how to handle their waiting lists. Certain principles apply.

- If a facility accepts someone on its waiting list, this is tantamount to declaring responsibility for the person. If the facility is not sure that it wants to do that, then it should set the duration (3 or 6 months) or number (25 or 50 names) allowed, and tell the patient whether he or she is on the list. If the patient does not make the waiting list, then he or she should be so informed and advised to contact other hospital or community resources, if available. Periodically, say every three months, the facility should reopen the waiting list and call those refused in order of their application. The facility hopes that at least some will have found other sources of help. If it is objected that all that the facility has done is to exchange one long waiting list for two shorter ones, I would reply, first, that the facility has accepted no obligation for the later patients; second, that it has left the responsibility for treatment with these patients and their physicians; and third, that it has a true active list, which it can then manage intelligently.

- If some triage is necessary before the facility accepts a patient for treatment, then the division will not be between the active and inactive waiting list, but between the urgent and the elective or less urgent. Again, it takes fortitude to say no, but facilities will need to decide to treat those for whom it can do most. At the same time, it needs to labour in the community to encourage and even resource other helping programs for those whose need, though real, is less. Classes and groups may be formed by community health agencies, service clubs or churches. The facility does no one any good by pretending to take responsibility for those it cannot care for. At the same time, all triage should conclude with a prescription of what the patients and their families can do to assist themselves.

A Service-Specific Strategy — Drug Utilization

Drug use evaluation (DUE) is the name of a formal prescription monitoring program that can be employed by a hospital or group of hospitals. In the program, a limited number of drugs is selected for monitoring. These will be drugs that

- are frequently prescribed;

- have a known potential for interaction or adverse drug reactions (ADR) in general, or in a particular population;

- will usually also be costly.

In conjunction with the pharmacy, the Pharmacy & Therapeutics committee approves a set of criteria for the prescription of these monitored drugs. After the criteria have been cleared by the medical staff, monitoring begins. All prescriptions of the drug are then monitored for the presence of the criteria. Prescriptions lacking the key criteria will be flagged for subsequent review by the P&T committee. Deviations will be brought to the attention of the prescribing physician.

Although the program is expensive to set up and, depending on the number of drugs monitored, costly to operate, it is claimed to be effective in changing physician prescribing practice, in enhancing the safety and appropriateness of drug therapy, and ultimately in lowering costs.

7.5
Outcomes
Management

The concepts of "medical uncertainty" and "small area variation" escaped out of the medical literature into public consciousness in Canada in about 1988. John Wennberg had been tracking the phenomenon of variations in the use of medical care in New England since the early 1970s. In a 1988 article he wrote:

> *Consider the following statistics. A resident of New Haven, Connecticut is about twice as likely to undergo a coronary bypass operation as is a resident of Boston; for carotid endarterectomy, the risks are the other way around. The numbers of knee and hip replacements per capita are much more common among Bostonians, while New Havenites experience substantially higher risks for hysterectomy and back surgery. The risk of hospitalization for Boston is substantially higher for a host of acute and chronic medical conditions, including back pain, gastroenteritis, pneumonia, chronic bronchitis, and diabetes, even though the residents of the two communities are very similar in demographic characteristics related to the need for care.*

> *These statistics illustrate the intellectual confusion in the heartland of scientific medicine. The residents of Boston and New Haven receive most of their care in hospitals and from physicians who are affiliated with some of the nation's finest medical schools. The practice styles in these communities have very different implications for costs, but the alternative theories about appropriate practice they represent have gone unchallenged or examined by academic medicine.*[24]

It was a short step to move from small area variation, that is, geography as a determinant of what care a patient will receive, to the question of the appropriateness of clinical choice. The Rand Corporation in California carried out a number of studies in which expert clinicians were asked, from the patient record, to judge the appropriateness of the medical decision taken. In one such study, the authors summarized their findings: "Inappropriate use varied by county from 8% to 75% for coronary angiography, from 0% to 67% for carotid endarterectomy, and from 0% to 25% for endoscopy." [25] In their study, *Appropriateness of Care,* Brook and Vaiana show a chart whose title reads, "Physician's Practice Style is Most Important Predictor of Caesarean Section Deliveries." [26]

It may be difficult for physicians, exposed to this literature for years and intimately familiar with the shades of grey that pervade much medical decision making, to fathom the amazement that such findings cause among the lay public. This insight was underscored for one Chief of Staff when he casually acknowledged to the chair of the hospital board that there were inappropriate procedures being carried out in the hospital.

There have been two answers to the problem of appropriateness. Practice guidelines, parameters, protocols are one; the other is outcomes management (OM). This is a multifaceted approach linked to the name of Paul Ellwood in Minnesota.[27]

Outcomes management hopes in the long term to amass a large clinical data base by patient condition. Data on each condition would show the variety of treatment modalities used by frequency and effectiveness. Effectiveness is measured by means of a functional questionnaire completed by the patient a relevant period after the intervention. OM intends two benefits. First, attending physicians would have access to the data base at the time when they are making clinical choices for the patient. The data base would tell them for each diagnosis (1) the variety of treatment modalities registered in the system by frequency, (2) their effectiveness scores, as registered by the patient questionnaires, and (3) any variation by age, sex and other patient features. The underlying hope of the system is to reduce medical uncertainty and improve physician choice by presenting relevant clinical experience at time of choice.

The other feature of outcomes management is relatively undeveloped. OM is intended to assist patients in making choices for themselves through production of videotapes in which the leading treatment options for a particular condition are portrayed in lay terms. In one such videotape on the treatment of prostatitis, two physician sufferers with the condition are interviewed. One had elected surgery, a prostatectomy; the other had chosen "watchful waiting". Both courses were described personally and from the perspective of clinical effectiveness. In showing these videos to an Ontario audience in 1990, Wennberg stated that quite a high proportion of patients who had initially elected to have surgery ultimately declined it following their viewing of the videotape. Apparently, there was no corresponding shift towards surgery among those who had not chosen it in the first place.

There are no immediate consequences of outcomes management for Canadian clinicians. The system needs to develop in both the building and accessibility of the data base (which incidentally is not intended to cover either all or most CMGs or DRGs, only the 16-20 that account for 80% of conditions requiring hospitalization). Meanwhile, the creation of videotapes suitable for patient viewing needs to proceed apace. There are two important underlying motifs, however: first, clinical choice based on wide experience may be a corrective to small area variation; and second, patient choice needs to be assisted by the full presentation of the major options.

References

1. The scope and variety of reports, including special studies, that can be obtained from HMRI are outlined in the institute's annual *Pricing Policy Guide.*
2. Ontario Hospital Association/Ontario Medical Association/Ontario Ministry of Health/Hospital Medical Records Institute (1988). *Guide for Hospital Utilization Review and Management in Ontario.* Toronto: OHA.
3. *Ibid.,* p. vii.
4. Canadian Council on Health Facilities Association (1991). *Acute Care: Large Community and Teaching Hospital, 1992.* Ottawa: CCHFA, Governing Body, Area VII, pp. 22-23.
5. Ontario Hospital Association/Ontario Medical Association (1990). *Prototype Hospital By-laws.* Toronto: OHA, pp. 65-66.
6. See Note 2; pp. iii-iv.
7. Ontario Hospital Association/Ontario Medical Association/Hospital Medical Records Institute (1991). *Guidelines for Medical Manpower Planning and Impact Analysis in Hospitals.* Toronto: OHA, p. ii.
8. Feferman, I. and Cornell, C. (1989). How we solved the overcrowding problem in our emergency department. *CMAJ* 140(1 Feb.):273-276.
9. Harrison, F.P. and Roger, W.F. (1990). Quality utilization management: Preliminary results to a Canadian approach. *Health Services Management FORUM* (Winter):28-33.
10. Catchpole, B.L. (1991). A utilization management success story. *Dimensions* 68(2 [Feb.]):16-17.
11. Langelle, P. (1987). Wetaskiwin physicians manage bed allocations. *Dimensions* 64(2 [Feb.]):28-30.
12. *Ibid.,* p. 30.
13. Catchpole, *op. cit.,* p. 17.
14. Lang, D.A. (1991). *Medical Staff Peer Review.* Chicago: American Hospital Association, p. 35.
15. *Ibid.,* pp. 54, 64.

16. Scarborough General Hospital (1990). Three years of physician bed management. *Agenda: The Newsletter for the Medical Staff 3*(3 [Sept.]):8-10.
17. Zander, K. (1988). Nursing case management: Strategic management of cost and quality outcomes. *JONA 18*(5 [May]):23-30.
18. *Ibid.,* p. 26.
19. See Note 16.
20. See Note 8.
21. Hassen, P.C. (1991). Continuous quality improvement: The experience of St. Joseph's Health Centre. *Canadian Journal of Quality in Health Care 9*(1[Nov.]):2-4.
22. Schurman, D.P. (1991). Continuous quality improvement: Perspectives and experiences of CEOs of Canadian hospitals. *Canadian Journal of Quality in Health Care 9*(1 [Nov.]):5-6.
23. Zander, *op. cit.* (see Note 17), p. 25; emphasis added.
24. Wennberg, J.E. (1988). Commentary: Improving the medical decision-making process. *Health Affairs* (Spring):99-106.
25. Leape, L.L., Park, R.E., Solomon, D.H., Chassin, M.R., Kosecoft, J. and Brook, R.H. (1990). Does inappropriate use explain small-area variations in the use of health care services? *JAMA 263* (5 [2 Feb.]):669-672.
26. Brook, R.H. and Vaiana, M.E. (1989). *Appropriateness of Care: A Chart Book.* Washington, D.C.: National Health Policy Forum, George Washington University. Chart 8, p. 9, citing Goyert, G.L. (1989), *NEJM* [16 March]:706-709.
27. Ellwood, P.M. (1988). Shattuck lecture: Outcomes management — A technology of patient experience. *NEJM 318* (23 [18 June]):1549-1556.

Part 3

Risk Management

8

Managing Risk in the Department

8.1
Risk Management and Quality Assurance

Risk management (RM) and quality assurance are complementary systems. While they do not have the same scope, they share important territory. At conferences and in the literature people sometimes engage in sterile discussions as to which came first and which is the more important. The truth is that each can be more important than the other in different contexts. This is because the systems have different but complementary purposes. The purposes of QA, as we have seen, are the continuous monitoring, improvement and accounting for the quality of performance. In contrast, RM is a comprehensive and proactive strategy to defend the facility and all its dependents from harm. RM may not make you well, but aims to keep you out of trouble; QA constantly strives for improvement, but is not naturally equipped to count the cost (as does utilization review and management) or notice the risks (as does risk management).

Let me illustrate the relationship between QA and RM. Bill was hired straight out of school and was seen to have great potential. He was given a thorough orientation to the job, but as he seemed slow to catch on, his supervisor, Mary, teamed him up for a week with one of the more experienced technologists. This seemed to work: Bill said that he felt more confident and thought he could handle his rotation on his own. However, before the end of his first solo week, Mary was hearing snide comments from other members of the department. She let it be known that Bill was new and she expected people to give him support and advice if he needed it. She did not hear anything further for a time, although she suspected that staff were still not happy with Bill. Then she started to hear complaints from the floors. After she persuaded one head nurse to document an incident involving a patient, she invited Bill into her office. They talked about the incident and the patient's attitude to him, apparently because of Bill's race. Mary made it clear that Bill was going to have to learn to cope with prejudiced patients and asked him if he had ever had an opportunity of working this through with a counsellor. With Bill's consent, she arranged a meeting with one of the social workers who counselled employees. About two weeks later, Mary returned to the department after lunch to learn that Bill had been involved in a fight and had given one of her staff a bloody nose. When she investigated the incident, she concluded that Bill was responsible for the quarrel and for losing his temper. She suspended him for three days without pay, with the warning of a more severe penalty should a similar infraction occur again.

In this story we see a supervisor take a series of steps in staff *development*: Bill's orientation, pairing him with an experienced buddy, supporting his integration into the team, providing counselling for a personal problem. But when he crossed the line into bad behaviour, Mary moved swiftly from staff development to *discipline*. She still hoped to have Bill as an effective long-term employee, but he had broken the rules. In this scenario, staff development represents QA

— the continuing effort to improve — while discipline stands for risk management — the need to act now to prevent further damaging occurrences. The topic is still Bill's future, and it is his behaviour that will decide the extent to which he is dealt with through one set of strategies or with the other.

In earlier discussions of the nature of QA, its scope was intentionally limited to the quality of service provided. RM comes into play only if the level of service provision poses a threat to hospital or patient or other. But RM is also concerned with all threats wherever they occur in the life of the facility, whether in client service, management/support activities, or in the enjoyment of the amenities of the facility. Slips and falls in the parking lot are as much an issue for RM as are medication incidents. RM is concerned with good order and freedom from threat, QA with improvement in client service. They meet, says Joyce Craddick, in the *adverse patient occurrence* (APO). We will revisit Craddick and APOs later.

8.2
Definitions

Risk management as a formal strategy or discipline has been practised by commercial ventures for decades. Companies have striven to lessen the number and severity of their accidents and occurrences in order to protect their assets and limit their exposure. Mechanical breakdowns, supplier failure, work stoppages, lawsuits and grievances, bad publicity — all can adversely affect a company's bottom line. Thus, risk management has had to grow to encompass all threats to the stability and profitability of a business. This basic history of the development of risk management has several implications for health care facilities.

- Although risk management is a discipline new to health care in the United States in the 1980s and in Canada in the 1990s, it has a long history and its own practices, language and forms, which health care must adopt. Hospitals have to operate in the same legal, commercial and insurance environment as do companies in other industries.

- Risk management is a comprehensive strategy and risk a comprehensive concept. Risk is not, as is so often supposed, simply liability or the threat of suit.

- Underlying risk there is the financial reality. Risk is always translatable into dollars and cents; it is not just threat or jeopardy. The probability of the occurrence and its potential impact are quantified so that the reality and severity of a risk can be assessed financially.

- Although risk management may be new as a formal concept to the organization, health care facilities will discover, as did commercial companies decades ago, that a wide variety of risk management practices are already in place, whether they are called infection control, radiation protection, or other names.

Commercial definitions of risk management identify threats to net property, income, liability and personnel.[1] In developing the first accreditation standard for RM in Canada, we added reputation and called the five exposures the *Risk Pentagon*.[2] We were particularly concerned to highlight risk to patients, in addition to personnel, although RM authorities may counsel that patient risk is assumed in the term "liability". In fact, we may want to draw a heptagon to illustrate a hospital's seven major exposures, because its responsibilities to the environment are being made more explicit in legislation and by public opinion. The Risk Heptagon CRIPPLE shows the hospital's major exposures as those of:

- *Customers:* its patients and families, and students

- *Reputation:* government and community relations

- *Income:* from all sources, for all purposes

- *Property:* the physical integrity of its assets

- *Personnel:* its major asset in a labour-intensive industry

- *Liability:* including all those matters that never come to suit, and

- *Environment:* the hospital's duty to act as a good corporate citizen.

The second definition, which will be the topic of this chapter and the next, is that of risk management itself.

Risk management is. . . a management system or process. It has four basic steps:
- *the identification of risk,*
- *risk assessment,*
- *taking actions to manage risks, and*
- *the evaluation of risk management activities.*[3]

We will examine in turn risk identification, risk assessment, actions to address, and the evaluation of loss experience. In this chapter our primary concern is the embodiment of these concepts in practical strategies within line departments. In Chapter 9 the focus shifts to the organization of risk management as a hospital-wide strategy.

8.3
The Identification
of Risk

This is the place to make the point that risk management is not a retrospective loss accounting system but a prospective or proactive loss prevention program. There is a good analogy with staff performance appraisal. Although in performance appraisal the employee and supervisor talk about performance in the year past, the purpose and focus of their meeting is the improvement of communications and performance in the future. So too with RM; and it is the identification of risk that makes possible its management in the future. You cannot guard against what you do not foresee.

Managers, i.e., department heads and head nurses, can identify risks germane to their areas by three means or from three sources: learning from past experience, learning from others' experience, and learning on the job. The first is retrospective, the last concurrent, and the second, both retrospective and continuous.

Learning from Past Experience

In spite of the absence of an organized facility-wide RM program there will be, as we have noted, all sorts of evidence of people managing risks. Over time departments have identified occasions on which their clients, personnel or processes were in special jeopardy and have instituted quality

Exhibit 8.1
Data Retrieval

QC Records	Event Records
Preventive Maintenance Records	Patient Incidents
Fire Inspection Reports	Employee Incidents
Narcotics Records	Medication Incidents
Laboratory QC Records	Infection Reports
Food Service QC	Patient Loss Records
Occupational Health and Safety Inspection Reports	Department/Unit Logs
HARP Inspection Reports (Radiology)	On-Call Reports
	Security Reports (thefts, break-ins, vandalism)

control procedures to address these special risks. Where it has not been possible to identify a special threat, they have made sure that random injurious events were recorded and reported. Departments need to retrieve both sets of data — the quality control records and event records — such as those shown in Exhibit 8.1.

The second source of past experience is personal. Managers should first answer for themselves the questions listed in Exhibit 8.2. Then they can see that all members of their department have an opportunity of responding to the same questions. Individuals can be interviewed; groups of staff can be asked to brainstorm the questions at a department or section meeting. Then some collation needs to occur. A report to staff of the findings of the exercise will likely yield further risks not discovered in the original inquiry.

Exhibit 8.2
Risk Identification Questions

---

1. In your department, what is the worst thing that could happen?

2. In your experience, what untoward events have occurred that were important because of their severity or frequency?

    (a) Severe event(s)

    (b) Frequent incidents

3. What times or situations make your operation most vulnerable to risk/loss?

4. What negative data have you had to act upon recently in QA or Occupational Health and Safety?

    (a) QA

    (b) OH&S

5. What special risks are identified in your professional literature?

Learning from the Experience of Others

The last of the risk identification questions introduces the second of the manager's sources. Learning from other people's experience is much less expensive than learning at one's own cost. The manager and her professional staff can do more than recollect; they can search for what is known about risks specific to their profession and departmental functions. If they cannot ask their hospital library to carry out a search of the literature, they can follow the steps suggested in Exhibit 8.3. Nor should they neglect their professional meetings and networks. There is in risk management no premium on originality. The advice is to find managers who have already developed their own profiles, and borrow shamelessly from them. If that is not possible, managers can look for one or more peers in other hospitals who will work with them on such a profile.

The reason I have described learning from others as being concurrent as well as retrospective is that risk exposures change both with clinical and technical advances and in society's values and expectations. Environmental integrity, patients' rights, and matters of consent are major issues of the 1990s hardly mentioned in the 1970s. Managers need to be prepared to incorporate into their department's risk profile new hazards identified by their colleagues and their profession's literature.

The object of learning from the past and from others is to assemble a *risk profile,* a listing of the special risks inherent in the work of the department. Many of the risks occurring on the department's long list of answers to the risk management questions will prove to be generic rather than specific. Some will be generic to patients. Because they are sick, patients are prone to slips, falls, misunderstandings, paranoia, unpleasantness, getting lost, and a host of other accidents — and not just in "my" department. Similarly, there will be environmental hazards not specific to the subject area and personal issues identified on the department's list, just because "people (staff and supervisors)

Exhibit 8.3
Steps in a Literature Search for Service/Professional Risks

1. The search is for literature that reports or discusses hospital *occurrences, incidents, claims, complaints,* or *misadventures.* Another descriptor is *adverse patient occurrences* (APOs). These occurrences are specific or relevant to the work of the department or service instituting the search.

2. The search could include literature within the last 3 – 5 years; information over ten years old may lack relevance.

3. Choose journals of your profession or specialty plus general hospital/clinical journals.

4. Identify sources where the indexes or literature may be found: hospital library, public library, university/faculty library.

5. Find in these places the relevant search tools, e.g., *Index of Hospital Literature, Index Medicus*; annual indexes in the last/first issue of each volume of specialty journals; on-line data bases such as the *Medline Data Base* and *Health Planning and Administrative Data Base* of the MEDLARS system.

6. Each data source will have its own arrangement. Check before attempting to use it.

7. Retrieve articles whose abstracts or titles most closely match the topic. Then seek other titles whose match may be less good.

8. Make notes of the salient features so that in a month's time the facts are still available to you.

9. Pull the search together with a simple two-page summary.

will be people." When these are segregated under those titles (Patients, Occupational Health & Safety, and Personnel) what is left is the raw material of the department's risk profile. Managers may choose to use their principal function and important component lists (see Chapter 2) as a format on which to arrange their risks. In using these lists, managers will unwittingly find themselves asking whether there are not risks — as yet unidentified — associated with the functions and components unaddressed.

I still have the notes I took when interviewing the administrative manager of a radiology department five years ago. My questions are lost, but the manager's answers I listed under the following headings: Harm to Patients, Misdiagnosis, Equipment (Induced Risks?), Risk to Equipment, Risk Attendant on the Use of Chemicals, and Use of QA (in Identifying Risk?). His answers appear in Exhibit 8.4.

Exhibit 8.4
Risks in Radiology Identified by Administrative Manager

1. **Harm to Patients**
    *   Anaphylactic reactions to contrast media — IVP reactions.
    *   Falls off table.
    *   Patient unattended can wander, vomit and aspirate, have seizures.
    *   Risk increases with elderly and ethnic patients. Now using language cards and getting high-risk patients to change in Emergency, where they can be observed.
    *   Risk of back injury to elderly during transfer on and off table.

2. **Misdiagnosis**
    *   Film incorrectly read or views taken did not show.

3. **Equipment**
    *   Locks and controls malfunction, camera or tube falls.
    *   Radiation hazard largely removed by routine HARP semi-annual inspection and preventative maintenance (PM). Full inspection when machines are moved or modified.

4. **Risk to Equipment**

   - $1.3 million CT: Its $500K computer could be cooked if improperly used or humidity/heat controls fail.

   - Damage to X-ray equipment, mobile unit, or radiation shield. Department has a 3-week orientation program for new employees.

5. **Risks Attendant on Use of Chemicals**

   - Contrast media, etc. and developing fluids.

   - Use of goggles and wash-up facilities.

   - Film processing chemistry (with auto-processing, no skin exposure).

6. **Use of QA**

   - PM program (1-2 days p.a. for thorough PM program) lessens risk of malfunction and radiation.

   - QC on processors reduces number of repeats.

   - Greater awareness of risks due to regular departmental and OH&S inspections.

   - Incidents are recorded: IV running dry, slips and falls. ("Near misses" are not recorded.)

   (End of interview.)

Participants in my QA course have taken this list and attempted to develop a risk profile from it. They have sorted the entries in various ways, but the most satisfactory method has combined the subject of the risk (patient, equipment, staff) with the features that have heightened their jeopardy (e.g., infirmity of the patient, inexperience or workload of staff, age of the equipment). One such arrangement is shown in Exhibit 8.5.

Exhibit 8.5
Identified Risks in Radiology Arranged in a Risk Profile

Risk	Factors Intensifying Risk
Harm to Patients	
• Anaphylactic reaction to contrast media	
• Falls off table; injury during transfer	Language problems
• Harm when unattended in waiting/change rooms	Patient illness/infirmity
• Patient irradiation	
• Trauma from equipment; failure of locks/controls	Age of equipment
Harm to Equipment	
• Improper procedure with CT scan causing damage	
• Failure of humidity/heat controls causing damage	Inexperienced staff using unsafe procedures
• Damage to X-ray units	
• Damage to portable X-ray	
Harm to Staff	
• Trauma from X-ray and other heavy equipment	Age of equipment
• Exposure to caustic chemicals	Shortage/inexperience of staff
Loss of Income	
• Failure to document and bill hospital out-patients	Inexperienced staff

Learning on the Job: The Concurrent Identification of Risk

In health care there are three well-known methods of reporting negative events as they occur: incident reporting (the most common method), occurrence screening (the most thorough and expensive), and occurrence reporting (something in between).

Patient Incident Reporting

Probably ninety per cent of Canadian health facilities operate a patient incident reporting system, in which all events that harm or threaten to harm a patient are recorded on an official form by the staff member closest to the event. Although these systems tend to be unpopular and are not overly productive as methods of risk identification, their major advantage to the manager is that they are in place. It is always easier to improve what is already working than to introduce something new that may not work or work as well.

Incident reporting systems are unpopular with staff because they require self-reporting and seem to imply some confession of guilt or blame. In addition, they are cumbersome; incident report forms, in multiple copies, often comprise six to ten sections on legal-size paper and may take considerable time to complete. In most hospitals, Nursing is the only department that reports incidents on a consistent basis.

Managers who wish to increase the usefulness of this system can help their cause by adopting three strategies. First, they can simplify the reporting process. It may not be within their discretion to change the hospital's incident report form, but they can devise a quicker way for staff to file a preliminary report or to report minor occurrences. For example, a manager might introduce a departmental log or diary or an index card report that would ask for the date, time, location, name of patient or staff affected, a one-sentence statement of what occurred, and the reporter's signature. If the manager or her deputy checked these entries daily they could determine whether the incident needed to go to the second stage, i.e., a full incident report. Second, managers can reduce the potential for guilt or blame by demonstrating concern for the reporter and focussing on the system that failed rather than the person at fault. Third, managers can show the value of incident reporting by the use they make of the information. Staff will appreciate feedback on numbers and types of incidents, and what they or the team can do to reduce their occurrence.

These suggestions are not merely pious. Braft, Way and Steadman describe how they were able to increase the volume and reliability of the incident reporting system of the New York State Office of Mental Health.[4] At one point in my career I was suddenly made responsible for "accident prevention" in a hospital that grossly under-reported its employee incidents. Instead of there being twenty incidents to each lost-time injury [5] there were only four or five, and many of the lost-time injuries were discovered only when the hospital or employee sought recovery from the Workers' Compensation Board (WCB). By increasing awareness, presenting reporting as a positive act (and failure to report a WCB injury as a heinous crime), and providing good and interesting feedback, we saw the hospital's reporting statistics double each month for three months, without an increase in lost-time injuries. It can be done.

Occurrence Screening

Occurrence screening is the concurrent reviewing of in-patient charts by a team of trained screeners who look for evidence of actual or potential patient occurrences. The screeners, usually health records staff or nurses, are given lists of specific or generic events which they are expected to recognize in the charts. Both the technique and the early generic screens came from the 1976 California Medical Insurance Feasibility Study (CMIFS). In this study, sponsored by the state medical and hospital associations to assess the feasibility of no-fault health insurance in California, a blue-ribbon panel of screeners (MDs and medical audit experts) reviewed 20 000 records from twenty-three hospitals against a list of twenty occurrences. One of the often-quoted findings of this study was that nearly one in twenty (5%) patients of the 20 000 was deemed to have suffered an adverse patient occurrence (APO), including 1% that "were determined probably to be due to legally recognizable fault on the part of the provider." [6]

There are many screens in use today; Exhibit 8.6 shows one of the earliest lists, which was derived immediately from the CMIFS. Many U.S. hospitals and consultants have developed concurrent screening programs; however, the best known is the Medical Management Analysis (MMA) System of Joyce Craddick, MD,[7] a pediatric cardiologist and one of the original CMIFS screeners. A good concurrent screening system aims to integrate quality assurance and utilization review with risk management by using comprehensive screens. In addition, these systems prescribe how potential occurrences discovered in the course of initial review are handled, so that professionals are not embarrassed by groundless challenges.

Occurrence screening is such an uncompromising and apparently complete system that it must be far beyond the scope of choice of an individual department. Hospitals that wish to consider it should be aware of its major strengths and weaknesses. Among its strengths:

- It combines effectively QA, UR and RM.

- It answers the basic problem of the clinical care provided by physicians, which most other QA and RM strategies neglect.

- It is concurrent. The patient in the hospital can benefit almost immediately from the recognition of a lapse in his or her care.

- It uncovers systems problems more reliably and much earlier than audit or other inquiry.

- It provides excellent, current and highly specific information on the quality of care for various audiences.

Exhibit 8.6
Outcome Screening Criteria: Acute-Care Hospitals

1. Admission for adverse results of out-patient management.

2. Admission for complication or incomplete management of problem on previous hospital admission.

3. Hospital-incurred incidents, including drug and transfusion reactions.

4. Transfer from general-care unit to special-care unit.

5. Transfer to another acute-care facility.

6. Operation for perforation, laceration, tear or injury of an organ incurred during an invasive procedure.

7. Cancellation of or repeat diagnostic procedure due to improper preparation of patient, technician error or failure.

8. Unplanned return to the operating room on this admission.

9. Unplanned removal or injury or repair of an organ or part of an organ during an operative procedure.

10. Myocardial infarction during or within 48 h of a surgical procedure on this admission.

11. Infection not present on admission (nosocomial).

12. Neurologic deficit present at discharge that was not present on admission.

13. LOS = 90th percentile.

14. Cardiac or respiratory arrest.

15. Death.

16. Other complications.

17. Subsequent admission for a complication or adverse effect of this hospitalization.

18. Subsequent visit to Emergency Room or out-patient department for complication or adverse result of this hospitalization.

— From: "Medical Management Analysis: A System for Controlling Losses and Evaluating Medical Care." (1978). Monograph. Toronto: Marsh & McLennan. Reprinted with permission.

There are disadvantages to every strategy. On the debit side of occurrence screening we must list three provisos:

- It is silent concerning non-clinical quality and risk. What is not in the chart is not available for review.

- It is costly. The demand to review every chart every 48 h or 72 h does not come cheap. Estimates for acute hospitals vary: one screener for every 50 beds or one per 125 beds,[8] 1.5 screeners per 500 discharges [9] or four screeners for each 1000 discharges per month.[10]

- Not every medical staff will buy into occurrence screening. Its very efficiency increases its threat to physicians who do not support peer review and resent what they may construe as management interference.

Few Canadian hospitals have adopted occurrence screening, probably because of its costs. But those who have, have been well pleased with their investment.[11] Toronto's Queen Elizabeth Hospital, having recognized the diminished time costs required in a long-term care facility, has implemented it — again, with real satisfaction.[12]

Occurrence Reporting

Occurrence reporting is a risk identification method whose best-known employer is the Chicago Hospital Risk Pooling Program (CHRPP). CHRPP is a trust that functions "as the professional liability insurer for 14 community general hospitals in the Chicago Metropolitan area." [13] The program has encouraged its members to monitor, trend and report defined risk occurrences in four high-risk areas:

- Operating room/recovery room (OR/RR);

- Labour, delivery and nursery;

- Emergency; and

- Surgical and non-surgical ambulatory care.

Exhibit 8.7
Generic Occurrence List: Patient Occurrences

1. Patient complaint.

2. Request to see someone outside the treatment system — ombudsman, lawyer, administration.

3. Premature or unauthorized discharge AMA.

4. Incidents of inadequate consent (uninformed, invalid or unsigned).

5. Medication treatment or test incidents, including procedures done on wrong patient, and patient refusal of medication or treatment.

6. Patient reactions — arrest, anaphylactic shock, seizure, dizziness.

7. Patient falls.

8. Other patient injury.

CHRPP used to require occurrence reporting in Intensive Care, but the low number of claims from ICU allowed the program to cease mandatory monitoring of these units.

Unfamiliar with CHRPP and the terminology of occurrence reporting, I proposed in 1987 what I called a Structured Incident Reporting System (SIRS) for implementation in a suburban hospital in Toronto. This hospital-wide program depended on the use of three generic incident (i.e., occurrence) lists dealing with Patients (Exhibit 8.7), Occupational Health & Safety (Exhibit 8.8), Personnel (since deleted), and one department-specific list (Exhibit 8.9). SIRS proposed that hospitals should introduce one occurrence list, after review and local modification, at a time over a three- to six-month period. Meanwhile, each department would be encouraged to develop its own specific screen with maximum staff input. The advantages of a hospital-wide occurrence reporting program are:

Exhibit 8.8
Generic Occurrence List: Occupational Health & Safety Occurrences

No Injury	1.	Environmental Hazard
	2.	Personnel Exposure
	3.	Faulty Equipment
Damage/No Injury	4.	Fire or Environmental Contamination
	5.	Equipment or Property Damage
Staff Injuries	6.	First Aid
	7.	Medical Aid
	8.	Lost-Time Injury
Client Injuries	9.	Patient/Visitor Injury

- It can be developed from a hospital's existing incident reporting system.

- The definition of occurrences tells everyone what they *must* report.

- The wide promulgation of generic lists and the staff-developed specific occurrences is intended to make reporting a universal requirement, rather than special to Nursing.

- Occurrences come readily coded (i.e., a slip or fall; a return to Emergency within 24 h).

- Occurrence reporting is inexpensive, non-punitive and non-threatening.

- Occurrence reporting is not restricted, either to the patient chart or to patient care alone. It will pick up incidents wherever they occur.

Exhibit 8.9
Department Occurrence List: Security Department

1. Theft or other loss of property.

2. Damage to property.

3. Unauthorized access.

4. Visitor injuries.

5. Misdemeanours and offences (incl. smoking incidents).

6. Threats to people or property.

7. Parking incidents.

Exhibit 8.10
Effectiveness of Risk Identification Systems[†]

System	Reporting Potential
	(% of Actual Occurrences)
Medical Management Analysis (MMA)	90-95%
Occurrence screening	80-85%
Occurrence reporting	40-60%
Incident reporting	5-30%

[†] By estimated yield of medically related adverse patient occurrences (APOs).

— American College of Surgeons (1985). *Patient Safety Manual,* 2nd ed. Cited by Craddick, J.W. (1986), "Medical Management Analysis in 1986," *in:* Chapman-Cliburn, G., ed. (1986), *Risk Management and Quality Assurance: Issues and Interactions.* Chicago: JCAHO, p. 72.

The drawbacks of occurrence reporting are, first, that the system must be reinforced with feedback to staff and be re-energized at least annually. Hospitals need to monitor and seek to maintain the quantity of occurrences reported. Second, occurrence reporting, while more effective in the identification of APOs than an incident reporting system, is significantly less effective than occurrence screening. The figures are shown in Exhibit 8.10.

The concurrent identification of risks has two purposes: risk management and damage control. However, the righting or rewriting of what *has* occurred are strategies inferior to managing the future, which is the goal of RM.

8.4
Assessing Risk

Assessment is the second of the four activities that constitute the risk management strategy. Risk assessment takes place retrospectively, prospectively, and concurrently at the departmental and corporate levels. In line with our current focus, this chapter will discuss only those activities that take place within the department. The matrix in Exhibit 8.11 sets out the various risk assessment functions.

Exhibit 8.11
Risk Assessment Matrix

	Concurrent	Past → Future
Departmental	Damage control	Risk profiling
Corporate	Claims management	Risk weighting

Initial Assessment

I am indebted to Paul Allen [14] of Marsh & McLennan for the important insight that the initial assessment of the risk event is made by the first witness(es). Allen has called the response of the witness "intuitive assesssment" as the staff member moves to aid the affected person or to protect people or things from further exposure to a hazard that has appeared. The staff member's mind processes quickly the questions of who or what is damaged and needs assistance, who or what is in jeopardy of further injury, what can be done immediately, and what help might be needed by the staff member to stabilize and remedy the situation. A second assessment takes place within the department when management reviews the incident and addresses the needs to report the occurrence and to involve corporate risk management. This review may occur within minutes, certainly within twenty-four hours. In the matrix shown in Exhibit 8.11 I have used the term damage control because this is the intent of staff in handling an incident at the time it occurs.

Risk Profiling

The more common purpose of assessment in RM within the department is what we have referred to earlier as risk profiling. This is the development of a picture of the jeopardy or risk that is specific to that department. The profile will include both generic risks — those common to most line departments — and special risks that are unique to the principal functions of the unit, area or department. The profile will be made up of all of those risks identified by the means previously suggested (incident reporting, occurrence screening, occurrence reporting). The profile, once developed, will remain fairly stable over time, although each new incident or new risk identified from external sources will challenge the shapes and shadings of the picture. There is one caution. Sometimes a department's very success in addressing major risks may blind management to the continuing hazard. For example, the major hazard of radiation exposure is routinely addressed by several layers of preventive actions, including quarterly inspections of the machines and their emissions, the use of radiation badges, special procedures and the wearing of protective shields and garments. The fact that the department's experience shows patient slips and falls to be its most frequent and serious type of incident must not blind management to its obligation to continue to address its major hazard.

The intent of risk assessment and particularly risk profiling is to see the enemy clearly enough to wage war against it. Risk assessment is the prelude to the management of risk.

8.5
Action to Manage Risk

Risk is managed in two ways: by risk financing and loss control. These strategies are not alternatives or substitutes for each other. Each major risk should be financed and, to the facility's best efforts, controlled. Risk financing is handled at a corporate level, and its examination will therefore be deferred to Chapter 9. This chapter will discuss the five standard loss control strategies — avoidance, referral, prevention, reduction, and segregation — as they apply to health care.

Risk Avoidance

Although usually not possible, the simplest strategy is to avoid altogether the activity associated with high or repeated risk. Insurance companies stop insuring certain types of risk, such as automobile insurance. Retail chains close stores that have repeatedly operated at a loss, and manufacturers terminate product lines for similar reasons. In health care a family physician may decide, because of his increasing age and that of his practice, to cease doing obstetrics. Sometimes hospitals have to close operating suites because of an inability to recruit anaesthetists. Both instances illustrate risk avoidance.

Risk Transfer

It is unusual for a health facility to be able simply to walk away from the obligation to provide a patient service. Instead they will refer patients to another facility and, in so doing, transfer the risk associated with the service to the new service provider. Because of the increasing sophistication of its biomedical equipment, one hospital's maintenance department contracted out the work — and thus transferred the liability for the reliable operation of the equipment to the contractor. A hospital laboratory, noting that it had low volume in an expensive test, decided to have the test taken off its laboratory licence and referred future tests to a medical centre lab. This is risk transfer.

Prevention

What used to be called accident prevention is the commonest loss control strategy and comes in several forms. It is *protection:* hard hats and safety boots, lead aprons, sharps boxes, vaccination; double-bagging infected linen; inspection of incoming software programs for computer viruses; the preadmission screening of patients referred for high-risk procedures so as to restrict the procedures to the patients best able to tolerate them. It is *preventive maintenance* and equipment standards: restrictions on the use of personal appliances; regular inspection of equipment and machinery; monthly fire equipment inspections; weekly running of back-up generators. Prevention is set *procedures* for such actions as the administration of medications; the checking of the crash cart; the hand-over of the surgical patient at the operating suite; the receipt of money; and the review of physician credentials. Finally, risk prevention is staff *education*. Procedures and protection in the manual do not prevent anything; they must be used and practised reliably. And simply "telling it once" is not enough in a hospital, where shifts change, staff move, teams re-form — and each time something is lost.

At a medical staff meeting six weeks ago, physicians began to discuss the charting of DNR ("do not resuscitate") orders. They all knew what to write, when and where to chart it, but their opinions had no consistency — they might have been from four different hospitals. The risks to life, liability, family happiness (not to mention the confusion and abuse to nurses on duty) were enormous. Risk prevention is a continuous effort to protect, prevent, prescribe, inform and train all those who can limit the risks and stop the incidents. This means that patients, families and students need to be enrolled on the side of safety by making them part of the processes of the hospital. On a non-smoking flight last year it was other passengers who noticed someone sneaking into the washroom with a cigarette and alerted the flight attendants. Patient participation in care and choices will increase their ability to prevent incidents that might involve them.

Loss Reduction

Following the publication of the CCHFA companion document on risk management,[15] we were criticized for listing loss reduction as an action to manage risk. Readers must decide whether to use this class of action in their risk management efforts. Avoidance, transferral and prevention are strategies that anticipate risk; loss reduction and asset segregation are efforts to minimize the effects of an incident at its occurrence.

Once an incident has occurred it is too late to stop it, but it may not be too late to ameliorate its effects. The response to a patient injury is medical attention, comfort and —

whatever the lawyers may advise — honest disclosure. When fire prevention fails, prompt fire procedures by all staff will usually save the situation.

A patient incident does not have to be serious before staff think about loss reduction. If patient satisfaction is as important a criterion of service as we — and CQI — say it is, then patient complaints should call it into play. Informed, confident and settled patients do better than those who are anxious and offended. But there is a second reason; patient suits are more often related to their sense of offence than they are to the reality of injury. One constant factor in patient suits against doctors and hospitals is a breakdown in communications. Risk management says that every patient complaint is an event calling for re-establishment of communication and the helping relationship.

Asset Segregation

The strategy here is best summarized by the admonition, "Don't put all your eggs in one basket." Important assets — financial, environmental, human, informational — should all be provided with back-up or divided systems so that jeopardy to one will not threaten the other. Back-ups for water and power supply, computer tapes, meals, boilers, equipment and personnel are necessary features of the modern hospital where the loss of one or more critical resource cannot be allowed to stop the operation of the facility or endanger its patients.

Putting It All Together

It is important for each department to make explicit what its risks are and how it is actively handling them. Exhibit 8.12 does this for Radiology, using the risk list developed by the department head in Exhibit 8.4 and reformatted in Exhibit 8.5. Exhibit 8.12 carries three columns: the risk, the generic strategy attempted (avoidance, prevention, etc.), and the specific action taken. The value of this kind of summary sheet is fourfold: (1) it identifies the risks under surveillance and management by the department; (2) it forces the department or unit to identify specifically and generically what it is doing; (3) it has the potential to show gaps in service or attention; and (4) it provides an essential backdrop to evaluation, in that new occurrences challenge the adequacy of both the department's risk identification and loss prevention strategies.

Exhibit 8.12
A Department Manages Its Risk: Matching the Risk Profile with Actions to Manage Risks

Risk	Strategy	Action
1. *Harm to Patients*		
Anaphylactic shock	P	Patient screening for allergies
	R	Availability of crash cart
Falls/transfer injuries	P	Patient screening (second RT aide, etc. with elderly/infirm)
	P	Use of language cards for ethnic patients
Patients coming to harm when left unattended	T	Stretcher in-patients must come with RN/RNA
	T	Sick infirm patients change and wait under observation in ER
Patient irradiation	R	Restriction of both dose and diffusion through correct procedure and equipment inspection
Trauma from equipment	P	Regular preventative maintenance
	$T	Outside contractors retain financial liability

Exhibit 8.12 continues on page 242

Risk	Strategy	Action
2. *Harm to Equipment*		
Damage to CT computer	$T	Regular maintenance by supplier
	P	Full staff orientation and testing
Damage to X-ray units	$T	Regular maintenance by supplier
	P	Preventive maintenance by staff
		Staff orientation
Damage to portable X-ray	$T	As above
	P	As above; special attention to moving gear-wheels, etc.
3. *Harm to Staff*		
Trauma from equipment	P	Regular supplier and preventive maintenance
Back injuries from moving pts. and equipment	P A	Annual staff training in body mechanics: lifting, pushing, etc.
Exposure to caustic chemicals	P	Safety procedures in use of chemicals
	R	Availability of safety equipment, goggles, wash-up facilities
4. *Loss of Income*		
Failure to document and bill	P	Orientation to registration procedure
	P	Data check on EDP system

Strategies: A = Avoidance   T = Transfer   P = Prevention
R = Reduction   S = Segregation $T = Indemnity clauses
with external contractors

8.6
The Evaluation of
Risk Experience

As with other aspects of the risk management strategy, risk evaluation is conducted at two levels: the departmental and the corporate level. The department's evaluation loops it neatly back into quality assurance and indicators.

In discussing indicators in Chapter 3, we labelled priority-one indicators "risk indicators" and recommended their regular collection, monthly reporting on a run or trend chart, and annual review. In carrying out this routine the department is involved in risk evaluation as surely as it is doing QA. The method of annual review recommended was the analysis of the data behind the indicator figures, by means of a focussed study. Departments will bring to these annual reviews special concerns arising from their involvement in risk management. In their examination of a key or leading indicator the department will look for trends and make comparisons between 1992's results versus those of 1991 or the department's goal or industry benchmark. In looking at risk indicator data the department may be less interested in overall trends than in the repetition of incidents against which specific RM action strategies had been instituted. The issue in RM is more than the comparison of performance. Each occurrence asks one of two questions: How did this happen in spite of the department's proactive remedy? *or,* Is this occurrence an isolated incident or one of a class which should be reviewed and addressed?

This second question may necessitate a return to QA. One of the four criteria mentioned in the QA *Standards* for the choice of indicators — or, for that matter, audits — is "problem-prone". A serious, yet apparently isolated incident could trigger an audit, one of whose purposes would be to ask, How likely is this sort of incident to recur? The physicians' discovery of the lack of agreement on the charting of DNR orders was a serious incident waiting to occur. The MAC should demand an audit to determine the state of the hospital's practice and seek follow-up action and a reaudit in three to six months.

In summary, risk evaluation in the department is (1) the monthly monitoring of risk indicators; (2) the annual review of the risk experience beneath the indicator, in light of the department's actions to address risk; and (3) the investigation of emerging risks in order to assess the need to employ new strategies.

References

1. For example: Head, G.L. and Horn, S. II (1985). *Essentials of the Risk Management Process,* vol. 1. Malvern, PA: Insurance Institute of America, pp. 10-12.
2. Canadian Council on Health Facilities (1991). *Risk Management for Canadian Health Facilities.* Ottawa: CCHFA, p.1.
3. *Ibid.,* p. 5.
4. Braft, J., Way, B.B. and Steadman, H.J. (1986). Incident reporting: Evaluation of New York's pilot incident logging system. *Quality Review Bulletin (QRB) 12*(3 [March]):90-98.
5. The industrial accident pyramid is 600 incidents to 30 lost-time injuries to one death.
6. Craddick, J.W. (1979). The Medical Management Analysis system: A professional liability warning mechanism. *QRB 5*(4 [April]):577.
7. *Ibid.*
8. Carlow, D. (1988). Occurrence screening can improve QA programs. *Dimensions 65*(6 [June]):20-22.
9. Nordal, C.A. and Ang, J.B. (1988). Occurrence screening in long-term care. *Dimensions 65*(3 [March]):23-27.
10. Joint Commission on the Accreditation of Healthcare Organizations (1990). *Primer on Indicator Development and Application: Measuring Quality in Health Care.* Oakbrook Terrace, IL: JCAHO, p. 78.
11. Carlow, *op. cit.* (see Note 8).
12. Nordal & Ang, *op. cit.* (see Note 9).
13. JCAHO, *op. cit.* (see Note 10).
14. Allen, P., personal communication.
15. CCHFA, *op. cit.* (see Note 2).

9

Corporate Risk Management

9.1
Taking Charge

When the CCHFA introduced quality assurance to Canadian health facilities in 1983 the Council told its audiences, quite correctly, that much or most of what it wanted to see on survey was already in place in the line departments of hospitals and other facilities. What it discovered early was that, more often than not, there was nothing of QA at the head of the organization. The same was true of risk management when the first Canadian *Standards* were published in 1990. Neither senior management nor the board were experienced in taking responsibility for risk. Often this is a matter of the way facilities are organized rather than evidence of neglect. Let me illustrate with a personal experience.

Before offering advice on risk management to a well-run community general hospital, I asked for the opportunity to interview senior management to ascertain what its members were already doing in RM. I started with the Chief Financial Officer, who handled all the placement of the hospital's insurance. His only complaint was that the insurer often did not tell him what claims it settled nor what it paid out on the hospital's account each year. The hospital's Vice President of Operations was responsible for the management of all claims and suits against the hospital. Nearly all of these were patient related; the more serious included physicians, and involved the VP in working for and with the hospital's Chief of Staff. The person in charge of the hospital's incident reporting system was the Vice President of Nursing, although incidents other than nursing were also reported. The Vice President of Human Resources had three risk-related systems reporting to her: the hospital's Occupational Health & Safety program (OH&S), the labour relations grievances, and the Security department. The Vice President of Plant Services had a watching brief over all the facility's environmental services and over contractors who undertook installation and renovation work. The two VPs in charge of Professional and Hospital Services had cognizance of risk events within the six or eight departments reporting to each of them.

Was this otherwise well-run hospital managing risk? Certainly it was responding to risk, but as for managing it — probably not.

Did the seven VPs communicate with each other and the hospital CEO on a regular basis? No; they communicated only on a need-to-know basis. For too long, people in health care have acted as if good hospitals, departments, and units — and, of course, staff — do not have occurrences or incidents. The perception is that incidents are avoidable; to talk about them is to wash dirty linen in public.

What should that hospital, and others similarly organized, do? Its senior management had one important principle straight: management were the ones who were concerned about risk and were therefore taking respon-sibility for it. But they needed first to become for RM what they are in their day-to-day functioning: a team that shares information, provides mutual support, and decides action.

Second, they wanted to move from occurrence accounting to the management of risks, from managing the past to anticipating the future. Third, they had to take seriously their responsibility to report RM to the board. This would expose their fourth need: for new or better ways to organize the hospital's risk information.

Many hospitals have reached this point and gone beyond, including probably the hospital whose story I have just recounted. I remember visiting another hospital about the same time where the senior management group was the facility's risk management committee. Once a month at its weekly management meeting it would consider RM reports of various kinds and review the status of the program. Today, when corporate staffs in hospitals have to reduce in size and cost, that hospital's method of managing its RM program has much to commend it.

9.2
Gathering All
the Reins

Health facilities entered the 1990s (and the formal opening of the risk management season) with a wide variety of risk-related activities programs and systems. These can be enumerated as follows:

1. Department-based risk management activities, whose quantity and effectiveness may vary widely.

2. A hospital-wide incident reporting system focussed chiefly on patient-related occurrences.

   Additional nursing reporting systems often include:

3. Medication-incident reporting, and

4. On-call reports or logs dealing with all manner of irregular events occurring on evening and night shifts, weekends and holidays.

5. The hospital's mandatory infection control program, which compiles monthly statistics and reports quarterly to the Infection Control committee of the MAC.

6. The hospital's Occupational Health & Safety program, mandated usually by provincial legislation.

7. Monitoring the volume and content of letters of complaint and commendation received by the Executive Office. In addition, many hospitals regularly poll current or former patients by means of a printed satisfaction questionnaire.

8. Activity reports from hospital Security. These will catalogue calls for assistance, parking incidents, and investigations into reported thefts, break-ins, vandalism and unsecured premises.

9. Emergency measures, such as fire drills and training, patient-search procedures, internal and external disaster planning and exercises, including call-in drills.

10. Quality assurance, related to risk management through its quality control elements and the monthly reporting of risk indicators.

11. The responsibility to report legal actions to the board.

Left out of account in this impressive list are two bodies of information: the handling of clinical risk by medical staff, and the hospital inspection programs of external regulatory agencies. Most of the latter were begun and continue today because of the risks underlying the functions inspected. Their importance in RM underlines the value of insisting that all external inspections be reported to senior management and the board as part of each department's QA program.

The MAC must function as the medical staff RM committee and its chair, the Chief of Staff, should sit as a member of

Exhibit 9.1
Quarterly Summary of Risk Management Events

Program/Department/System: _____

RM report for 3-month period ending: _____

1. Total incidents   This quarter: _____

                         Last quarter: _____

                         Same quarter last year: _____

2. Breakdown: No. of incidents involving

    (a) Patients _____ (b) Staff _____

    (c) Others _____ (d) Property _____

3. Effectiveness: No. of incidents thought to be addressed by current RM strategy _____

4. Severity: No. of incidents referred to Claims Management _____

5. Listing of severe incidents by type:

    _____

    _____

    _____

    _____

Date _____ Signature _____

                        Title _____

the hospital's senior management in its RM capacity.

How does the CEO or designate gather all these reins into his or her own hands? Probably the first essential is to make sure that all these activities are reported to members of the cabinet. All that needs to be known should be known to anyone seated at the senior management meeting. Second, the facility will do well to establish a generic report form (see Exhibit 9.1) for use by these independent systems or programs. The executive needs to know the following facts from those reporting:

- The *total number of incidents* per quarter (comparative figures for the last four quarters could be helpful);

- *Subtotals of incidents* for patients, staff, other people, and property;

- *Effectiveness:* the number of incidents thought to be addressed by specific RM action;

- *Severity:* the number of incidents referred for claims management; and

- A listing of *severe incidents.*

Third, each program (particularly those numbered 5, 6, 8 and 9 in the ten-item list, page 248) should be expected to submit an annual report on its activities and experience. This requirement of programs is underutilized in hospitals and benefits both the program, which must then carry out an annual stock-taking, and senior management, which receives substantial information in a year's perspective.

9.3
Risk Management and Accreditation

Having outlined the need for risk management and methods by which management can take charge, we need to step back and examine the requirements for RM in the current (1992) accreditation *Standards.*[1] There have been some substantial developments in the *Standards* since their introduction in the 1991 edition.[2]

References to RM in the Accreditation Standards

Responsibilities for risk management are prescribed for two groups in the facility: the governing body (GOV) and administration or management services (MGT). Standard VIII in both sections is titled "Risk Management".

Risk management occurs four times in the *Standards* for Medical Services (MED), and is described as a "principal function" of Medical Services (MED I, 2.1). Risk management is listed as one of the facility-wide activities in which Medical Services should be represented and participate (MED II, 7). Risk management is further listed as a possible topic in new medical staff orientation (MED V, 1) and the source of information for medical staff development (V, 2).

For most departments, risk management will occur in Standard II (7.3) as an accountability of the director of the service, in Standard III (1.1) as a topic for department policies and procedures, and in Standard V as a topic for new orientation and staff development (1 and 2).

Definition of Risk Management

Risk management is described in both Governing Body (GOV VIII, 1.1) and Management Services *Standards* (MGT VIII, 1). The four-step process includes risk identification, risk assessment, actions to manage risks, and evaluation of risk management activities. The risks to be guarded against include those "to patients, staff, visitors and property of the facility" (GOV VIII, 1).

The Role of the Board

"The Governing body is accountable for the management of risks to the patients, staff, visitors and property of the facility" (GOV VIII). The risk management standard for the governing body (GOV VIII) has four requirements:

- The board is expected to *adopt a policy* for facility-wide risk management, in line with the definition already described. It is reminded that such a concerted effort will have cost implications. Thus, the policy must anticipate questions of spending and staffing priorities in the tight budgets of today's health facilities.

- The board is required to *receive reports* of risk management activities at least on a quarterly basis. The Council does not prescribe how this should be accomplished but does suggest some mechanisms that boards may wish to consider. These mechanisms include the involvement of a risk management committee and/or other committees that can receive and review "reports from management; reports from medical staff; reports from patient, family and staff satisfaction surveys; [and] correspondence from patients/families and the community"(GOV VIII, 2).

- The board is expected to *provide feedback* "on the results of risk management activities to management, medical staff and other staff."

- The board is expected to *monitor and evaluate* the facility-wide risk management activities. This requirement combines the fourth element in the risk management process — evaluation — with the sense of a comprehensive review: the demand that it be done annually.

In these reviews the board will consider the facility's activities, including those of its own risk management committee and other committees and structures within the facility. It may review questionnaires or surveys and consider other reports. In an annual or comprehensive review the board will be interested to compare activity with actual loss experience in order to judge the effectiveness of the risk management endeavour.

The Role of Management

"Management develops and implements facility-wide risk management activities" (MGT, VIII). This Standard holds management responsible for carrying out the risk management policies adopted by the board in:

1. Developing and implementing the system;

2. Adopting the four-step risk management process;

3. Identifying the individual risk management responsibilities of each service or program;

4. Developing and implementing RM policies and procedures;

5. Receiving reports (from the responsible services or programs) on a regular basis;

6. Doing the staff work necessary for the board's appraisal of the facility's management of risk and ensuring that the corrective action required is, in fact, carried through effectively;

7. Communicating to services or programs the evaluative comments and messages from the board; and

8. Co-ordinating all those activities related to risk, safety and quality, through communication, consultation, concerted action and participation. Specifically cited in this mandate are the following linkages:

   - *reporting risk management activities through the mechanisms established for quality assurance;*

   - *ensuring cross-representation on committees concerned with quality assurance, risk management and occupational health and safety;*

   - *using insurance claims and/or incident report data in selecting topics for focussed studies; and*

   - *amalgamating risk management and quality assurance within one service/division.*[3]

RM and QA: Integration or Differentiation

The "linkages" listed (MGT VIII, 7) recommend a different organization of RM than that proposed in this chapter. The Council calls for the complete integration of QA and RM, including joint reporting. I recommend a different integration and separate reporting routes.

It is essential that at the level of the department, management's demands for information be integrated, whether they be for Occupational Health & Safety, risk management or quality assurance. Department heads have only so much time and are reporting the one continuous experience of their department or unit. However, others may wish to code or differentiate their data later. The carrying of risk indicators within QA meets this principle. But certain risk events cannot wait for the monthly QA activity or the department's quarterly report. Instead they have to be fast-tracked, acted upon and reported to the QA/RM function immediately.

Similarly, the monthly reports of indicators will be forwarded to both the department's superior and QA/RM. The latter may simply file them until the month of the department's quarterly report to the QA committee. However, the department's vice president should monitor the run chart of risk indicators monthly for the sake of peace of mind and for discussion with senior management, acting as the facility's RM committee. QA has times and seasons; RM often demands accelerated responses — hence our differentiation in reporting routes.

The matter of the united QA/RM function will be discussed below, with reference to risk assessment and staffing.

Chapter 8 outlined the four activities at the departmental level that make up the risk management process: identification, assessment, action and evaluation. Here we need to examine the same activities as they occur at the corporate level.

9.4
Corporate Risk Management Activities

Risk Identification

There are four features of risk identification that are particular to the corporate level: the processing of external information, the choice of a concurrent reporting system, the reporting of medical incidents, and the handling of patient complaints.

External Information
Hospital management will receive undifferentiated information from a variety of sources: coroner's reports, claims statistics from an insurer, RM newsletters, product advisories from Health & Welfare Canada, notifications from equipment manufacturers, advisories from the provincial hospital or health association, as well as facility inspection reports from CCHFA, the provincial Departments of Labour and Health, the local fire department and others. The responsibility of management is to route this information to the relevant department and insist on a response, first as to its relevance to the department's operation (Do we in fact have this kind of equipment or product in use?) and, if relevant, the department's action. Management will carry out the same routing and response procedure for internally generated information such as patient questionnaires, complaints and commendations, reports from Security and OH&S inspections.

Choice of a Concurrent Reporting System
Although the three basic options — incident reporting, occurrence screening, and occurrence reporting — were

outlined in connection with departmental RM (Chapter 8), choosing among them belongs to the management of the facility. Whatever their choice, the effective operation of the reporting system will depend on all participants understanding and complying with the following:

- The purposes of incident reporting;

- The hospital's definition of an incident;

- That guidelines exist to specify under what circumstances an incident report must be completed;

- Who is responsible for making an incident report;

- That the completed incident reports follow a tightly controlled routing path, are kept confidential, and are inaccessible to all but authorized persons;

- The types of corrective action that can be generated by incident reports, and the understanding that this corrective action is generally non-punitive.

- That incident reporting plays a significant role in the prevention of medically related patient injuries, and that it can therefore help improve the quality of care and reduce the risk of malpractice claims.[4]

The Reporting of Medical Incidents

Doctors should be bound by the same obligations to report medical incidents and occurrences as any member of the hospital staff. Although there are structured situations in which this does occur, such as the Operating and Delivery suites, doctors do not generally believe that it is their business to report their own or a colleague's mishaps. What can be done?

Some suggestions:

- The CEO and chiefs of department must communicate to other physicians and hospital staff — mainly nurses and pharmacists — that they need to know and will treat all information confidentially for the reporter and sympathetically for the physician.

- This need to know must be communicated directly to health records professionals who must review each in-patient chart with insight in order to code and abstract its data. Many health records administrators are understandably reluctant to bring discordant data to anyone's attention. A list of occurrences reportable from the completed record is given in Exhibit 9.2.

Exhibit 9.2
Occurrences Discoverable by Health Records Analysis

1. Unplanned removal, injury or repair of organ during surgery or delivery.

2. Unplanned return to OR or delivery room.

3. Cardiac or respiratory arrest.

4. Transfer from general care to special care area.

5. Postoperative development of neurological deficit not present on admission.

6. Operative/procedural consent (including consent for ECT) incorrect or missing.

7. Admission within 7 days of discharge, same or related diagnosis.

8. Death.

9. Autopsy rate.

10. Self-inflicted injury.

11. Discharge against medical advice (AMA).

12. Unplanned in-patient admission following same-day surgery.

13. Caesarean section.

14. Development of decubitus ulcers among in-patients.

15. In-patient falls resulting in injury.

16. Patient-involved medication incidents.

- All complaints about physician performance will be screened carefully by a designated MD to see whether there is a *bona fide* issue before the physician is questioned.

- Medical leaders need to insist that risk management is neither surveillance nor the blunt end of medical discipline, but a physician support program. RM, if operating effectively, is a fail-safe system for physicians, catching their mistakes before they become liabilities, and identifying procedures that are unsafe and systems that are hazardous.

- On the other hand, incidents that, on investigation, demonstrate a serious performance problem must be documented in the physician's file. The Chief of Staff documents for the advice of the Credentials committee. The CEO is always informed.

Handling of Patient Complaints

In his *Loss Control Bulletin* (April 1989), McKerrow addressed the need for set policies on the handling of patient complaints:

> *The need for such policies and procedures is so evident and straightforward that it is hard to understand why Boards and Administrators have not universally developed them. At a recent conference on medical malpractice, participants were told that "at least 70 percent" of lawsuits were caused by physician attitude and communication failures!* [5]

One of McKerrow's concerns was that, without clear policies, neither board nor management had any right to expect that patient complaints would be handled sympathetically and promptly or be reported up the line.

What do clinical staff think of patient complaints? Those complained about hate them; they find them threatening and offensive. They also find it hard not to censure the complainer. Those who receive complaints about others hate them too. Complaints are a hot potato no one with any sense wants to carry. In the face of this widespread attitude, management needs to understand (and convey to staff) that patient complaints have three aspects: they are a call for help, a gift, and a warning.

- *A call for help.* Patients are not their normal selves. They are anxious, stressed and often stripped of their social support systems. Their complaints may not be informed, appropriate or realistic, but the patient wants help and needs understanding.

- *A gift.* It is the Japanese, in their continuous quality improvement, who say that a mistake, an error or complaint is a gift because it helps them to an insight about their process(es) that they had not seen before. So too in health care, there is the need to focus not on the threat to the individual clinician, but on the process that is flawed — and the possibility of its improvement.

- *A warning.* "At least seventy per cent of lawsuits were caused by. . . attitude and communication failure," says Dr. Curtis L. Cetrulo.[6] There must be very few serious claims or suits that were not preceded by warning shots, aggrieved shouts, cries for help, *if only* someone had taken them seriously.

Some prescriptions for management:

- Insist on the place of patient satisfaction data in the QA program of all clinical departments.

- Ask for the documenting of all patient or family complaints, including those given verbally. The old idea that "If it wasn't in writing, it need not be taken seriously" is a bad old idea.

- Call for the reporting of and response to all patient complaints within an immediate time frame (same shift, same day or within 48 h for those who have left the hospital).

- Route all client complaints received by the CEO and board chair to the risk manager, who will then take up the complaint, work it through with client and staff, and report its resolution to management.

Risk Assessment

Risk assessment at the corporate level means three things: claims management, the management of RM information, and weighting or costing of major risks or categories of risk. The material on the first two topics first appeared in the CCHFA companion document.[7]

Claims Management

CM is a specialist activity and one of the principal functions of a designated risk manager. Incidents or events thought to be severe, and carrying within them the possibility of complaint or suit, need to be handled immediately, reliably, confidentially yet in concert with essential parties. Claims management breaks down into a series of activities.

Recognition

The incident must be identified and its severity appreciated so that risk management can assume responsibility for the facility's defence against any possible claim. Late claims, or the notification to the facility of events it had not identified, are hard to defend. Risk management needs to know within 48 h if evidence is to be gathered and records secured. The person or department identifying the incident may recognize its severity and refer it to risk management, or it may be picked up in the course of daily review of incident or occurrence reports. It should be the rule that one copy of *all* incident reports, including those handled in organized programs, be designated for risk management and sent to that office.

Notification of insurer

The insurer should know as soon as possible about potential claims, and may have pertinent questions and advice that will assist in its immediate handling and investigation. A full written report will be filed later. This is more than a courtesy: failure to notify the insurer may affect coverage.

Gathering evidence

As soon after the event as possible, the claims manager will gather and secure as much evidence as is necessary and relevant to determine the facts of the case. The types of material that should be gathered include: the original copy (or a dated photocopy) of the patient's/resident's complete chart, all documents not normally considered part of the chart (fetal monitor strips, care plans), X-rays, pathology slides, equipment involved in the occurrence, the names and phone numbers of witnesses, the patient's/resident's roommates, and the names of staff on duty. All of this information should be placed under lock and key.

Discouraging claims

The facility, in co-operation with the insurer's assigned solicitor, should make considered response to the patient/resident or family in order to discourage them from launching a formal claim. (This may be of little use if they have already launched one.) It is no secret that open and honest communication tends to defuse tensions and eliminate previous miscommunication that often causes expensive and protracted litigation. Success at this stage will be encouraged or may have been doomed by the immediate response of staff in mitigating the loss or treating the injury *when* it occurred.

Investigation

A detailed and objective investigation of the claim should take place as soon as possible after the event. The investigation may start by ensuring the accurate completion of an incident report if one has not already been completed. Following this, staff involved in the incident should be interviewed and their statements recorded. Staff should be assured that the facility will help them and will provide them with legal advice if necessary. They should be cautioned about speaking with others, aside from the insurer's lawyers and facility management, about the incident. The facility should ensure that corrective actions are implemented as soon as possible to prevent an escalation of the damages or a repeat incident.

Working with the insurer's adjuster or solicitor
The facility should be careful to work with the assigned professional in each of the foregoing steps. In addition, a solicitor may become involved in directing such processes as preparing a statement of defence, examination for discovery, undertakings, trials, appeals, settlements, etc. Claims managers will become familiar with the essentials and routines involved in all of these manoeuvres; as they are usually carried out under the instructions of the solicitor, further description here is unnecessary. No adjuster, however expert, can achieve a timely and favourable settlement if risk management and facility staff have lost the case in their handling — or neglect of — the essential first steps: recognition, notification, gathering evidence, and investigation.

Risk Management Information System
In spite of all our best efforts incidents will occur, and they will occur in the best-managed facilities. When they do occur they will be addressed, post-incident, by loss reduction strategies, active investigation and claims management. It is one thing for an incident to occur; however, it is quite another when a similar or related incident recurs. Its repetition demonstrates that the risk has not been managed effectively. It also calls into question whether the facility has the capacity to recognize and learn from its own experience. This capacity to recognize and learn is represented in risk management by the facility's risk management information system (RMIS). A fully functioning RMIS should provide the following services to the facility's program:

- *Accounting.* The basic function is to collect, collate and report all risk incidents occurring during a given period.

- *Trending.* The system can demonstrate or deny the existence of trends in the data. If incidents are coded in various dimensions (type of incident, character of subject, place, etc.) then trending can be observed in all of those fields.

- *Costing.* Most incidents will be entered without cost data, but the field should be left open to accommodate financial information or a severity code.

- *Analysis.* The RMIS should have the capacity to provide an analysis of all similar incidents occurring over a given period so that the management of the attendant risks can be addressed in an informed way. The development of specific criteria for persons undergoing potentially high-risk procedures would be useful for preadmission assessment.

- *Claims tracking.* Because claims can occur at any time after an incident, subject to the interpretation of statutory limitations, and their handling can be drawn out over an extended period, it is important that the RMIS have the capacity to show which claims are outstanding, and which stage each has reached. Financial data will be an important part of this record.

For an RMIS to function effectively, the first essential is that data on all incidents reach the system, if possible as soon as the incident or occurrence is reported to someone outside of the department or unit. The system can register incomplete data and issue a demand for more at a later date. Second, the RMIS will function most effectively if incidents are recorded on forms that make the reporter code or categorize the event. For example, the originator may be required to identify the subject, type of incident, type of fall, as well as patient status and so forth. It is presumed that the RMIS has an interactive capability, which will allow it to register and report trends or recent repetitions for the event being recorded. For this reason early entry of incident data should signal trends-in-the-making or suspicious repetitions. Defective sutures, contaminated batches of medication, equipment malfunctions have in the past been detected by an RMIS flagging the repetition of related incidents.

It should not be necessary for any facility to create its own computerized RMIS; insurers and others are familiar with Canadian systems which work on a personal computer (PC). It is recommended that the risk management data base be handled by a dedicated PC. This will allow for high confidentiality and unrestricted use by those authorized access to the system.

Risk Costing

In most situations there is little question as to whether the facility should act to manage risk and finance possible losses. The action is automatic: if you can identify a risk, you should address it. But need a facility turn every accident or incident report into an action strategy? Or a companion question: In addressing risks, which do you decide to act on first? Risk costing is an important step in assigning priorities within the RM program. It depends on the simple equation:

Risk = Probability x Impact

The dollar value placed upon a given risk is the average cost of settlement multiplied by the estimated frequency of its repetition. Estimated frequency is expressed as a decimal or percentage — 2% or 0.02. With more common risks, hospitals may have figures for both their costs and frequency. Usually they will have to consult the literature: RM newsletters and analyses of claims generated by major insurers in Canada and the United States. Eustace and Sheridan [8] advise the use of a Probability/Impact Matrix (Exhibit 9.3). This matrix can be used with quite preliminary figures for both probability and impact, because its purpose is to identify risks that fall into quadrants B ("act now") and C ("continue to monitor").

Exhibit 9.3
The Probability/Impact Matrix

Impact

	Low	High
High	A	B
Low	C	D

Probability

— Eustace, D. and Sheridan, D. (1991). *Health Care Risk Management: A Home Study Course for Health Care Professionals.* Toronto: Ontario Hospital Association, p. 66. Reproduced with permission.

Actions to Manage Risk

All decisions on risk financing will be made at the corporate level, and corporate agreement will be necessary for risk control strategies that involve outside agencies. Both actions will be reviewed here.

Risk Financing
Risk financing is one of two essential strategies in a corporation's management of risk. It is not an alternative to, but a companion of, the various risk control actions discussed in Chapter 8 and revisited below. Undergirding all staff activities to reduce exposure and prevent accidents will be a financial safety net to cope with those incidents that were not anticipated or that penetrated the control shield so carefully constructed. Risk financing strategies fall into two groups: those in which the facility retains the financial obligations, and those in which it transfers such obligations to another organization.

Risk retention options

1. A facility can and probably will finance minor claims and repairs from its *current account*. Patients' belongings and prostheses get mislaid; equipment, whether personal or hospital, breaks or stops functioning and needs to be replaced. From a purely *financial* viewpoint, these small charges are seen as an ordinary cost of doing business.

2. For larger damages and claims, a facility may set aside a *funded reserve* out of which payments can be made.

3. Alternatively the reserve can be unfunded, which sounds like a contradiction. If it cannot fund such a reserve itself the facility can depend on a prearranged line of credit, so that it can *borrow* in order to pay off the losses incurred.

4. Many facilities have the option of participating in a captive insurance fund or subsidiary. Individual provinces in Canada operate *self-insurance* programs for their health care and social service facilities. In addition, there is a multiprovince insurance reciprocal in which facilities can participate. The essential difference between these programs and commercial insurance is the ownership of the funds. In self-insurance the funds and liabilities belong with the members. For this reason, self-insurance programs themselves usually carry commercial insurance for claims over a certain amount — $1 million or $3 million.

Risk transfer options

5. *Commercial insurance* is the most familiar option because nearly all adults in our society hold insurance policies on their automobile, home or life. So too must hospitals participate in insurance for the wide variety of their liabilities and obligations.

6. The last financial strategy is that of *transferring* the financial risk to another corporation. Head calls this strategy "contractual transfer for risk financing" to differentiate it from transfer for risk control. He explains

it as "transfer (under contract provisions often called 'indemnity' clauses) to an entity not an insurance company, of the financial burden for a loss." [9]

Risk Control Activities

While exposure avoidance, transfer, accident prevention, loss reduction and asset segregation all occur at the level of the department or unit, the choice of decisions and the determination to see them implemented occur at the corporate level. Thus senior management needs to recognize these strategies and encourage their consideration and employment within the organization.

Head and Horn [10] have devised a system of steps to take in risk management decision making. I reproduce these steps here as Exhibit 9.4 because they effectively summarize the RM process at the corporate level. Head and Horn combine assessment (which they call analysis) with identification as a single step and then provide three further steps en route to taking action to address risk. Their final step — monitoring and improving the risk management program — is what I term evaluation.

Exhibit 9.4
Steps in Risk Management Decision Making

Identifying Exposures to Loss

Identification

Types of Exposures
Property
Net income
Liability
Personnel

Methods of Identifying
Standardized surveys/Questionnaires
Financial statements
Records and files
Flow charts
Personal inspections
Experts

Analysis

Organizational Objectives
Profit
Continuous Operation
Stable earnings
Growth
Humanitarian concerns
Legal requirements
Significance
Loss frequency
Loss severity

Examining Feasibility of Alternative Techniques

Risk Control to Stop Losses

Exposure avoidance
Loss prevention
Loss reduction
Segregation of exposures (separation or duplication)
Contractual transfer for risk control

Risk Financing to Pay for Losses

Retention
Current expensing of losses
Unfunded reserve
Funded reserve
Borrowing
Captive insurer
Transfer
Commercial insurance
Contractual transfer for risk financing

Selecting Apparent Best Technique(s)

Choosing Selection Criteria

Financial criteria
Criteria related to other objectives

Decision Rules Applying Criteria

Risk control
Risk financing

Implement the Chosen Technique(s)
> Technical decisions
> Managerial decisions

Monitoring and Improving the RM Program

Purposes
> To assure proper implementation
> To detect and adapt to changes

Control Program
> Results standards
> Activities standards

— Head, G.L. and Horn, S. II (1985). *Essentials of the Risk Management Process*. Malvern, PA: Insurance Institute of America, p. 9. Reproduced with permission.

Action in the Medical Dimension

Somehow it is difficult to see that Head and Horn address the most serious and expensive losses that can afflict a hospital — medical misadventures. There are neither generic or simple answers. When Jessee addressed this problem he listed eight steps that are reminiscent of the Four-Legged Table of Chapter 5: credentials, QA, medical staff rules and leadership were his prescription:

> *If, in fact, providers are to be successful in controlling medical liability losses, they must develop a more comprehensive program that strengthens quality control mechanisms and heightens clinicians' awareness of their role in avoiding malpractice liability. Eight specific steps can be taken to reduce the risk of patient injury.*[11]

In order, Jessee's eight steps were:

1. Develop improved credentialing procedures;
2. Improve privilege delineation;
3. Create linkages between quality assurance and privilege renewal;
4. Increase understanding of the risks of hospitalization;
5. Enforce medical staff rules and regulations;
6. Appoint strong department chairs;
7. Support the actions of department chairs;
8. Improve accountability between medical staff and trustees.

Evaluation

Evaluation at the corporate level means two things: completing the loop and weighing the cost-benefits of the program. Board and management will go through the same cycle at their level that managers go through at departmental or unit level. They will use the events and losses that have occurred to test the adequacy of the RM shield that was erected to prevent them. This is to complete the loop. They will be aided in these comparisons between containment and escape by two factors: data that are presented graphically, and comparisons of their experience with industry norms. Reason insists that there must be lists of such norms — postsurgical infection rate, complication rates for different procedures, etc. — but I have yet to find them. Self-comparison may sound a poor alternative, but it has two benefits: the comparison is appropriate, and the data are quite adequate for the quest for improvement as distinct from the external validation of performance.

But how can the effectiveness of the program be judged? In about 1976, as a neophyte in the field, I attended the annual conference of the Industrial Accident Prevention Association (IAPA) at the Royal York Hotel in Toronto. Its program was stacked with North American gurus. The message I took back to my hospital was that there was no demonstrated correlation between accident prevention activities and accident rates, but that we must all nevertheless persevere in AP activities. My first response was disillusionment, but my second was a sense of security, in that neither I nor the hospital's program could be blamed directly for a bad year or a serious event. Rather, we should redouble our efforts.

If management is to evaluate its facility's RM program, as indeed it should, it can look at three features. The first is obviously settlement costs and incident rates. In an enterprise where one claim may result in a settlement of $1 million or more, the bottom line will tell you little about the effectiveness of the program either this year or in the year of the event. Instead, management will focus its attention on the subtotals: the hospital's WCB account, the cost of minor claims and out-of-court settlements, and of course the number and types of incidents that caused these expenditures. The second feature that should be examined is program activity: What have you done for me lately? RM should compile an annual report that will account for costs and describe activities such as complaint investigation or claims management, the implementation of corrective actions, the organization of drills (fire, evacuation, internal disaster) and education programs for staff and management. The third feature is participation. In the CCHFA companion document we use the expression "Every staff member is a risk manager." [12] Although responsibility for the risk management program must be grasped firmly by board and management, the best defence against loss is an aware staff. RM should be asked to show evidence of wide staff awareness and involvement.

9.5
Staffing

It would be unrealistic in Canada in 1992 to conclude the presentation of risk management with a large bill for staff, space and equipment. The costs of regulation that escalated in the 1980s are already resented by both physicians and management. Thus, those hospitals that have not invested in RM personnel are unlikely either to wish or to be able to do so in the foreseeable future. On the other hand, risk management is demanded by accreditation and, following the *Prichard Report*,[13] will be expected by the courts.

The key question is: What needs to be done in RM that cannot be done by department heads and others? For example, ninety per cent of quality assurance activities are carried out within line departments and clinical programs or specialties. What in the RM requirements cannot be decentralized? I believe there are three items:

1. *Claims management.* There must be few activities in a hospital that have such a direct effect on the bottom line. Every claim avoided and defence buttressed with relevant and contemporary evidence means less money paid by the hospital and its insurer. Claims management, which begins with incident investigation and carries through all the steps in litigation, is not for amateurs. One person needs to do it and do it often enough to do it well, serving line staff, the injured party and the hospital's interests. This is the reason why this person should also be the hospital's complaints officer.

2. *Data management.* Incident or occurrence reports need to go to one office and be entered on a system, probably a dedicated personal computer, so that the hospital can learn from its experience. Similarly, external information should go to one office so that its applicability can be assessed and messages passed on to those who could be

affected. Without a central processing office, the hospital's ability to anticipate and thus guard against risk will be crippled. For that hospital, RM will become a system of loss accounting.

3. *Education and management support.* Maintaining high staff awareness and participation demands a year-round program including orientation, staff development, and an RM week. New managers need early coaching in the hospital's RM system. The risk manager — if the hospital has chosen wisely — will also be the right hand of the Chief of Staff in organizing and maintaining RM activities at the clinical level. This latter responsibility requires dedicated expertise rather than time and willingness.

Many hospitals have solved their staffing problem by changing the title of their QA Co-ordinator to QA/RM Co-ordinator. My own prescription is to change the QA Co-ordinator's title to Risk Manager alone. There are two arguments to make in favour of this proposal. First, the requisite model of QA which I have proposed needs no dedicated staffing; in fact, dedicated staffing has tended to increase the management component, which we want to extract from the hospital-wide QA program. Second, RM is a new dish, not QA leftovers with a fresh sauce. If the QA Co-ordinator is not given a new title with a new job description, the employing hospital will get a willing worker but not a competent specialist, which is what all constituencies urgently need — board and management, medical staff, line departments, and the hospital's insurer and legal counsel.

9.6
Special Risks Associated with the Care of the Elderly

Those who work in long-term care are sensitive to the fact that so much seems to be written and done for acute facilities while little is addressed to them. Instead, they are expected to extrapolate what is relevant and translate it into their milieu. A fair criticism. It is important, therefore, to insist that risk management is just as much for chronic hospitals, nursing homes, homes for the aged and home care programs as it is for acute facilities. There are particular risks associated with the care of the elderly which deserve recognition and special management. Otherwise ordinary risks that can be fatal to the elderly include:

- Falls and fractures,

- Urinary tract infections,

- Flu, pneumonia, upper respiratory infections, and

- Choking.

Other sources of risk to the elderly:

- Cognitive impairment,

- Freedom to wander,

- Over-medication,

- Aggressive behaviour,

- Infirmity — loss of strength and balance,

- Food-borne hazards, and

- Decubitus ulcers.

These lists underscore the need for active risk management programs in all facilities and by all agencies caring for Canada's aging population.

References

1. Canadian Council on Health Facilities Accreditation (1991). *Acute Care, Small Community Hospitals.* Ottawa: CCHFA.
2. The text of much of Chapter 9, Section 3 is taken from: Canadian Council on Health Facilities Accreditation (1991). *Risk Management for Canadian Health Care Facilities.* Ottawa: CCHFA. Chapter 9, Section 4 is amended in the light of the 1992 *Standards.*
3. *Ibid.,* p. 28.
4. Orlikoff, J.E., Fifer, W.R. and Greeley, H.P. (1981). *Malpractice Prevention and Liability Control for Hospitals.* Chicago: American Hospital Publishing, pp. 74-75.
5. McKerrow, L.W. (1989). What happens at your hospital when a patient complains. *Loss Control Bulletin 11.* Ottawa: ENCOM Management Services, p. 2.
6. Quoted in *ibid.*
7. Canadian Council on Health Facilities Accreditation (1992). *Risk Management for Canadian Health Facilities.* Ottawa: CCHFA, pp. 31-35.
8. Eustace, D. and Sheridan, D. (1991). *Health Care Risk Management: A Home Study Course for Health Care Professionals.* Toronto: Ontario Hospital Association, p. 66.
9. Head, G.L. (1986). Updating the ABCs of risk management. *Risk Management 33*(6 [Oct.]):54.
10. Head, G.L. and Horn, S. II (1985). *Essentials of the Risk Management Process,* vol. 1. Malvern, PA: Insurance Institute of America, p. 9.
11. Jessee, W.F. (1986). "Preventing Malpractice Losses: Strategies for Hospital Medical Staffs." In: Dreuth, M.R. (ed.), *The Corporatization of Health Care Delivery: The Hospital-Physician Relationship.* Chicago: American Hospital Association, Chapter 7, pp.65-75. (Passage cited in text appears on p. 68.)
12. CCHFA (1991), *op. cit.,* p. 44 (see Note 2).
13. Prichard, J.R.S. *et al.* (1990). *Liability and Compensation in Health Care.* Toronto: University of Toronto Press.

Part 4

Continuous Quality Improvement

10

Continuous Quality Improvement

There are several terms in quality assurance that are virtually synonymous: the earliest was simply quality improvement (QI); next — particularly in Japan — came total quality control (TQC). Because in Western industry "quality control" has its own, different meaning, the term in North America became total quality management (TQM). The Juran Institute advocates strategic quality management (SQM); and the term now most commonly used in health care is continuous quality improvement (CQI). All of these terms refer to "a structured system for creating organization-wide participation in planning and implementing a continuous improvement process to meet and exceed customer needs."[1]

10.1
A Company
Reorientation

Some years ago I was called upon to examine the relationship between the medical staff of a teaching hospital and the
hospital's board and management. What surprised me was
the extent to which the university and its Faculty of Medicine
dominated the thinking of the hospital's physicians. The
hospital was just a venue, a clinical site, whereas the faculty
was the focus of the doctors' professional aspirations. This
situation is similar to that found in many hospitals. Health
professionals join the hospital to provide patient care, to
practise their clinical arts and skills. But before too long
organizational matters (assignments, teams, professional
distinctions, promotions, space allocations, staff and budget
issues) all become more important than the constant,
ordinary and repetitive flowthrough of work — in-patients,
out-patients, new and old patients, tall and short patients,
grey patients, no-name patients.

Continuous quality improvement is a system that encourages entire corporations to refocus on the value of the work
itself. From individual departments on upwards through the
organization, CQI causes everyone to scrutinize what happens
on the front line and to focus on the single question: How
well are our practitioners meeting the customers' needs?

CQI turns the organizational chart upside down and
acknowledges that the work of the front line is the most
important work of the corporation. CQI orients the entire
corporation to the customer, the ultimate recipient of all the
company's efforts. Historically, CQI has been embraced as a
corrective to poor quality, a solution to dwindling markets.
Sometimes, it has beeen advocated as a means of corporate
survival.

10.2
The Fundamental
Importance of
Process

In the spring of 1989 I received a call from the QA Co-ordinator of a hospital where, a year earlier, I had installed its QA program. Did I expect to be in her area soon? She had just returned from a QA program in Boston that had been a revelation, and she wished to tell me about it.

The program turned out to be one of the early courses on CQI mounted by the Harvard Community Health Plan. The QA Co-ordinator sat me down and talked to me for an hour or more about *process.*

She told me that everything that is done in an organization is achieved by means of a process or system — whether testing specimens in a lab, preparing food, or admitting a patient. And one intrinsic aspect of every process — whether it manufactures widgets or heals people — is *variation.* No ten successive widgets spat from the same machine are the same; no three, six, twelve tennis balls from the same lot bounce to the same height.

If the process is stable, the variation will occur randomly about a mean, and fall between an upper and a lower control limit (UCL and LCL), which can be calculated mathematically. The *common cause* of the variation is the process itself. So if you wish to correct what is happening you must change the process, not simply try to address the variation. Of course, sometimes there are *special causes* for variation, unrelated to the process itself. These are recognized by readings that occur outside the control limits ("outliers") or in the occurrence of trends or cycles in readings that defy the randomness of variation.

My colleague/mentor then related these concepts of process, variation and common and special causes to what we both knew about quality assurance. QA can be faulted in three respects:

- It tends to focus on individual performance: what the nurse does, or the mistakes the nurse makes.

- It attempts to correct outliers without any appreciation that the standards are arbitrary, and that these occurrences may well lie within normal variation for a given process.

- QA usually targets particular aspects of performance rather than the effects of the whole process.

In summary: QA promotes worker blame, meddling, and particularism.

It was probably that afternoon when I was also introduced to CQI's 85/15 rule. This is a rule of thumb that states that 85% of the error in any performance is *process* (or *common cause*) *error,* and less than 15% is attributable to *special causes,* including worker error.

This belief has three consequences. The first is obvious: that companies who are serious about quality must examine their processes rather than scapegoat their workers. Second: they need to find and implement strategies to improve their processes. Third: their best asset in process improvement may well be their workers, who are the experts in practice and can distinguish between systems that do and do not work.

---

10. 3
Continuous
Improvement

My conversion to continuous quality improvement is a long and personal tale. I include it because I believe that anyone who wants to understand CQI and appreciate its difference from earlier approaches must start with the concept of process and Deming's experiment of the red beads. (See Exhibit 10.1.) People who buy into CQI because of their excitement with worker empowerment, their belief in the customer and their desire for quality may not be around at the end of the day. They will have sworn allegience to yet another new and seductive trend that is probably brewing even as I write this.

Exhibit 10.1
Experiment: The Red Beads

This is a simulation that Deming includes in all his four-day courses, in which he sets worker-volunteers a task of producing batches of fifty white beads. The task is simplicity itself: With a specially designed wooden paddle that has slots for just fifty beads, participants scoop up one load at a time from a bucket containing 4000 beads. But 20% of the beads are red and, try as the workers will, these blemished products occur in every load in random numbers. Deming assists his workers with encouragement, exhortation, criticism, threats and despair — but all to no avail. Neither he nor the workers can overcome the faults in the process which they must operate. The process is more powerful than the motivation or manual dexterity of any member of the group.

— Adapted from: Walton, M. (1986). *The Deming Management Method.* New York: Putnam, pp. 40-51.

W. Edwards Deming, the incomparable living legend of quality improvement, was introduced to process and variation by Walter Shewhart, a physicist and statistician at Bell Telephone Laboratories in New York during the 1930s. Shewhart not only demonstrated the properties and behaviour of a process; he developed a system for improving processes. Shewhart, who fathered statistical process control (SPC), advised that processes were improved by a cyclical sequence in which the agent of change, having studied the process thoroughly, planned an improvement, tried it on a limited basis, checked the results or measured its effect, then acted to modify the process in line with the successful trial or to refine the experiment, before recycling with a new plan, new trial, reassessment, and action.

This *plan-do-check-act* (or PDCA) cycle, which Deming named after Shewhart, looks fairly obvious — just garden-variety trial-and-error. But such an assessment overlooks the scientist's relentless quest for better and better performance. The rotation of the cycle for Shewhart and Deming — and later, the Japanese — did not stop. It is intended to be a *continuous* improvement cycle. The PDCA cycle is the universal method of introducing improvements into a stable process. The Japanese still call it the Deming cycle because he introduced it to them in 1950.

But this discussion so far begs the question of what is meant by improvement. It will help to illustrate improvement strategies by means of an example.

10.4
A Hospital
Example

The manager of Physiotherapy has been alerted to the problem of waiting time for in-patients in her department. There have been complaints from the nursing units, and she has frequently noticed patients stacked up in the waiting room and adjoining corridor. In consultation with her staff, she establishes a standard of twenty minutes as the time within which in-patients will be seen, and arranges for the receptionist to note the patients' time of presentation and time of admission for treatment. The therapists agree to make a special effort to be prompt and expeditious in their treatments, without hurrying their care. At the end of the first week, the manager looks at the elapsed times for the seventy in-patients seen in the department over five days. (See Exhibit 10.2.) Twenty-one cases (i.e., 30%) showed elapsed times longer than the standard. In five cases the wait had been thirty-five to forty minutes, nearly twice as long as the standard allowed. The manager, in line with normal QA practice, went after the outliers. She discovered the following:

- *Six* of the cases were attributable to the patients' arrival in the department fifteen minutes or more before their scheduled appointment.

- *Six* cases all occurred on one afternoon when one therapist was off sick and her case load was divided among the other four.

- *Seven* cases were related to individual therapists' circumstances. One had to answer a *stat* call to ICU and consequently went over the standard with her next two patients (2 cases) before she caught up with her appointments. Two therapists worked significantly slower than the others and by the end of the afternoon were so off-schedule (5 cases) that their colleagues had to take their unattended cases to clear the department by 17:00.

The manager determined that she would let the head nurses on the two medical floors know that their patients were being brought down too early. She reasoned that she could not do too much about sickness or *stat* calls, but she decided to work with the two slower therapists.

Had the manager been working in a CQI hospital, her approach would have been very different. First, she would not have *done* anything. She and her team would have studied the process. Were the outliers special cause error or, more likely, common cause (supposing that the process were stable)? Next, she would not write off causes attributable to other departments, such as the nursing units, because they are a vital part of the patient-to-treatment process. Third, she might be chary of judging as special causes such

Exhibit 10.2
Distribution of Waiting Times for 70 In-patients in Physiotherapy, 1992.03.13

		Range	Frequency
0	3,4,5	1 - 5	3
	6,6,6,6,7,7,7,9,9,9,10,10	6 - 10	12
1	1,1,1,1,1,2,3,3,3,3,3,3,4,4,4,4,4,5,5,5	11 - 15	20
	6,6,6,7,7,8,8,9,9,0,0,0,0,0	16 - 20	14
2	1,2,2,3,3,4,4,4,4,5	21 - 25	10
	6,7,9,9,0	26 - 30	5
3	2	31 - 35	1
	6,6,7,7,8	36 - 40	5
			70

Mean = 17.1 min
Departmental standard = 20 min

occurrences as *stat* calls and staff sickness. Both may be common enough events to require allowance from the process. Fourth, before addressing the "faults" of the slow therapists, she may recognize that the scheduling system needs to take account of the variations in time required for different treatments, different patients and, yes, even different therapists.

But we have not disclosed the fundamental difference between the manager's actions under QA and CQI. In QA, when the manager is acting in the quality control mode, she will set standards and maintain adherence to them by addressing outliers. In CQI, when the manager is aware of the necessity (or opportunity) to improve performance, she is taught to improve the whole process. The intended result is that *all* patients will be seen more quickly, rather than that all will be seen within a fixed time. In Exhibit 10.3, Manager A is seen to address the leading lip of the bell curve, whereas Manager B is seen to raise the height of the bell and move it down the scale — i.e., creating heightened uniformity around a lower mean waiting time.

Exhibit 10.3
Improvement Strategies in QA and CQI

Manager A (QA) addresses outliers (shaded area) — occasions beyond the standard of 20 min

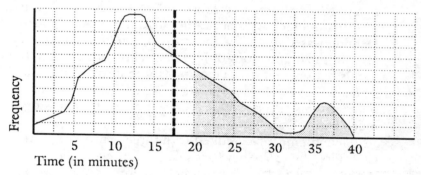

Manager B (CQI) addresses *all* occasions, controlling these variations and moving their mean (from 17.1 min) to 10 min (see new bell curve)

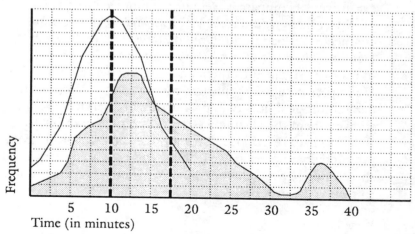

10. 5
The Power of Quality

Those who find value in names and origins will acknowledge Walter Shewhart as they come to understand process and variation, and begin evolving their own strategies for quality improvement. When introducing an audience to CQI, I always tell the bittersweet story of Dr. W. Edwards Deming, who shares much with our earlier hero, Dr. E.A. Codman. Deming was a prophet without honour in his own country. He laid the foundations of Japan's quality revolution in the 1950s but was not discovered by U.S. industry intil 1980 — when he was 79! I refer readers to Mary Walton's excellent book[2] on this prophet of our century, as she tells his story much better than I can.

Deming must be credited with three contributions to CQI. First, he took Shewhart's work on process and improvement to Japan, which became for twenty years the seedbed of CQI/TQM.

Second, he realized that if the owners and chief executives of companies were not committed to quality, quality control would remain the arcane art of the industrial engineer, as it had in the United States. On 13 July 1950, Deming dined with twenty-one CEOs from Japan's leading industries. "I talked to them an hour," he wrote in his diary. He impressed upon them the urgent need to select as their paramount goal quality in production and service. He showed them the (Deming) Chain Reaction (Exhibit 10.4). But the chain reaction is also a loop, in that the profit from productivity improvement (link 3) and increased market share (link 4) gets reinvested in quality improvement (link 1) to restart the process.

Wrote Deming:

I told them they would capture markets the world over within five years. They beat that prediction. Within four years, buyers all over the world were screaming for Japanese products.[3]

Exhibit 10.4
The Deming Chain Reaction

Improve quality

↓

Costs decrease because of less rework, fewer mistakes, fewer delays, snags, better use of machine time and materials

↓

Productivity improves

↓

Capture the market with better quality, lower price

↓

Stay in business

↓

Provide jobs and more jobs

— Deming, W.E. (1986). *Out of the Crisis.* Cambridge, MA: MIT, p. 3.

10.6
The Customer
as Participant

Deming's third contribution was to integrate the customer
with the production process. Everyone recognizes that there
is an ultimate customer. Deming's conviction was that the customer wishes to be written into the production process, not
just at the end as the eventual recipient or beneficiary, but
through the customer's response to the product as chooser
(or refuser) and employer of the good or service. This consumer
response should be sought and documented and looped back
into the improvement of the existing planning or of the new
product. (See Exhibit 10.5.) This was a revolutionary idea in
1950; some people in 1992 have still to catch up with it.

Exhibit 10.5
The Deming Flow Diagram

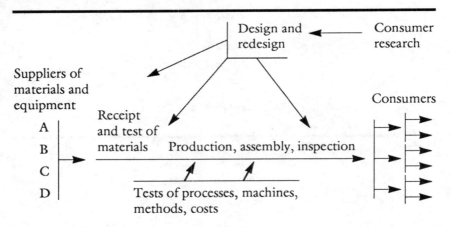

— Deming, W.E. (1986). *Out of the Crisis.* Cambridge, MA: MIT.

Deming's further insights into the customer are also fundamental to quality improvement. He stressed that satisfying the customer's immediate needs is not enough. The quality-conscious company should accept the responsibility of anticipating what the customer is going to want and need in three to five years.

And what of the production worker who never sees the customer or, for that matter, the finished product? Ishikawa's answer to steelworkers in Japan in 1950 was "the next process is your customer." [4] Interfacing processes, or departments, should see themselves and each other as customers and suppliers, not as enemies.

This chapter concludes with an addendum reviewing Deming's Fourteen Points for quality improvement. A mixture of the beliefs and admonitions of this acerbic yet gentle man, they make an interesting historical document in their own right.

10.7
TQM —
A Thought
Revolution in
Management

In spite of Deming's recognition that the quest for quality, pursued too low in the organization, would simply degenerate into the development of powerless specialists, and his efforts to gain the commitment of Japan's leading CEOs, Ishikawa remembers the early 1950s as

> *a period of overemphasis on statistical quality control. . . . Help was obviously needed at that time. Fortunately, Dr. J.M. Juran responded to the invitation of JUSE [the*

Japanese Union of Scientists and Engineers] *and came to Japan for the first time in 1954. He conducted seminars for top- and middle-level managers, explaining to them the roles they had to play in promoting QC activities.*

Dr. Juran's visit marked a transition in Japan's quality control activities from dealing primarily with technology based in factories to an overall concern for the entire management. There is a limit to statistical quality control which has engineers as its prime movers. The Juran visit created an atmosphere in which QC was to be regarded as a tool of management, thus creating an opening for the establishment of total quality control as we know it today.[5]

Juran's visit, however, is more important to CQI/TQM than just an interesting historical event. There is an international predisposition among senior executives, especially CEOs, to believe in quality if someone else will take responsibility for it. Like the frightened Old Testament prophet they answer the call, "Lord, here am I. Send him." To which Deming and others reply: "If *you* cannot come, don't send anyone else."

If quality is as powerful and effective in transforming the future of a company as TQM advocates insist, then why should executives show less personal interest in it than they would in the company's financial statement? The balance sheet is history from which people can make some predictions, but product quality is contemporary and is the company's future.

TQM practitioners would take us farther. They insist that when a whole company takes seriously its customers and the quality of its goods and services, this improves the quality of management and, consequently, the company's values and relationships.

According to author and lecturer Morris Massey, our behaviour as adults follows patterns established in childhood. Once the developmental mould is hardened, let us say beyond our teens, we will play out future situations as we learned in our formative years, unless we are seized by a "significant emotional event." [6] We can use the same analogy for a company. Once it has learned to operate within patterns based on the values and powers that have been legitimized, the company is highly resistant to change. And quality is a non-political goal — it thrives in cells rather than systems, which are the natural domain of politics. Thus it is relatively powerless.

There are two consequences of this sobering insight. Senior management must continue forever to legitimize quality — the quest for it, and the virtue of mistakes made in its pursuit. Second, it takes at least five (some would say ten) years to transform the culture of an organization in favour of quality. Throughout that time the forces of resistance, compromise and inertia will be ever present, threatening to erode the gains that have been achieved.

10.8
The Seven Pillars of Quality Improvement

We are now in a position to identify what I call the Seven Pillars of continuous quality improvement.

- An understanding of *process* and variation

- The continuous *rotation* of the improvement cycle

- An *obsession* with quality

- The centrality of the *customer*

- *Executive* reinvestment in continuous improvement

- *Staff* respect, empowerment and education

- The use of the *scientific approach*

These are listed in the order in which they occur in this chapter and historically. The first pillar — *process* — is also the memory aid to the Seven: *process, rotation, obsession, customer, executive, staff,* and *scientific method.*

In examining the historical development of CQI, we have already discussed the first five pillars. I would now like to address the last two, which have come to us from the Japanese.

General Staff and Quality Improvement

When quality improvement focusses on the process of production or service and comes to terms with the inevitability of variation, it puts the spotlight on management: those who choose and buy, create and authorize the process that workers must use. If the 85/15 rule is correct — i.e., that 85% or more of production or service errors are caused by the process, while less than 15% can be attributed to worker error — then that emphasis is justified. Workers are the victims of bad processes (including bad management), not their cause.

One of the most convincing proofs of this truth arises from investigations into medication incidents — errors made by nurses in administering medications on the ward. Studies show that when using a traditional medication system (in which the medications are drawn or poured from labelled bottles), nurses made between 5.3 and 20.6 errors per hundred. With unit-dose systems, the error rate falls to between 0.64 and 3.5 per hundred.[7] In a situation in which the performance of the *same* nurses was measured, first under a traditional system and later after the introduction of unit doses, their error rate dropped from 13% to 1.9%.[8]

We can go farther: Workers are fundamentally on the side of quality. Workers wish to take pride in and derive satisfaction from their jobs. When it comes to quality improvement, workers are the natural leaders because they know how their processes work, and the situations when they don't. What they need from management is the encouragement to address their problems and the authority to do something about them.

I give credit for this pillar to the Japanese because, from the earliest days of quality improvement, the Japanese Union of Scientists and Engineers (JUSE) provided education to staff. In April 1962 it began publishing a journal on QI especially for foremen, and later it encouraged the education of people on the shop floor through the QC Circle movement. (See Section 10.9, Structuring Quality Improvement.) Annual conferences for QC Circles began in 1963. The following year, Ishikawa wrote:

> *As of December 1983 there were 173 953 QC Circles and 1 490 629 Circle members registered with the QC Circle Headquarters. . . . My guess is that there are ten times as many circles currently in operation that are not registered.*[9]

Adds Imai: "One of the features of the Japanese workers is that they use their brains as well as their hands."[10] According to Eiji Toyoda, chairman of Toyota Motors, "Our workers provide 1.5 million suggestions a year, and 95% of them are put to practical use."[11]

The Scientific Approach

There is the nice admonition in CQI: "In God we trust — all others bring data." One of CQI's outstanding features is that it not only urges improvement but provides the tools to bring it about. QA has been criticized, quite appropriately in my judgement, for leaving department heads on their own when their data are poor and the need for remedial action is clear. Without particular management support, extra resources or new strategies, they have been expected to "fix it" — or at least to show data to indicate that they have!

Dr. Kaoru Ishikawa has been called by his compatriots "the founding father of the TQC movement."[12] His name is linked today with the cause-and-effect or "fishbone" diagram, one of seven basic tools developed by him and his colleagues in the JUSE in the late 1950s. These Seven Tools,[13] each of which will be discussed in detail in Chapter 11, include:

1. Pareto charts

2. Cause-and-effect diagrams

3. Stratifications

4. Check sheets

5. Histograms

6. Scatter diagrams

7. Graphs and control charts

These tools are put into the hands of the workers and are seen to be effective in solving 95% of the improvement problems that occur.

Two aspects of the use of statistical tools deserve comment. The first is the discipline that says that experience and gut feeling are not enough. If improvement is desired, the first step is to take seriously what is occurring now — to observe, study and measure it. These tools allow teams to study their processes and display their data so that diagnoses and remedial strategies are easier to find. As teams move into the improvement cycle — PDCA — the *check* stage is a return to measurement and analysis. Second, by putting the tools in the hands of the quality improvement teams (and the workers themselves), CQI sends the signal that improvement is reserved neither for the specialist, nor the industrial engineer, nor management. One interesting discovery in CQI is that the cost of process improvement rises in direct relation to the seniority of the person or group resolving the problem.

Exhibit 10.6 outlines the Seven Pillars of CQI along with their chief exponents. It should now be clear to the reader that CQI is much more than a performance improvement, or

Exhibit 10.6
The Seven Pillars of Continuous Improvement

Contributor	Principle	Memory Aid
Walter Shewhart	An understanding of process and the inevitability of variation	Process
Walter Shewhart	Process improvement is accomplished through the continuous rotation of the PDCA cycle	Rotation
W. Edwards Deming	The power of quality to transform a company's future High quality —> Low costs —> High productivity —> Low price —> Strong markets	Obsession with quality
W. Edwards Deming	The customer as a participant in production and design	Customer
Joseph M. Juran	Top management must begin the quest for quality and continually reinvest themselves in it	Executive reinvestment
Union of Japanese Scientists & Engineers	Quality improvement is accomplished by a staff that is well led, well educated and well respected	Staff respect
Kaoru Ishikawa	Continuous improvement depends on data derived from the use of tools of measurement and analysis	Scientific approach

quality enhancement tool. Both Ishikawa and Imai credit Juran with bringing company management within the purview of quality improvement. Before Juran, management's role was to hold the coats of more junior staff as they improved performance in production, sales and service. After Juran, management needed to improve the customer orientation of its own efforts and the actual performance of management systems. This is the meaning of the word "total" in the term TQC.

CQI is a proactive or prospective strategy. Everything about it is future oriented, from the heavy investment with which it begins, to the motivation of line workers in wanting to improve the processes they own.

10.9 Structuring Quality Improvement

For a short time in the early 1980s, Quality Circles were all the rage. They were, we were told, the reason for Japan's phenomenal success in manufacturing. I have in front of me Philip Thompson's *Quality Circles: How to Make Them Work in America*.[14] What is fascinating about this ten-year-old book (written to introduce an improvement structure that failed abysmally) is how modern and relevant it is. It mentions the seminal NBC documentary, "If Japan Can, Why Can't We?" (24 June 1980) and lists as training topics material we will review in Chapter 11: the problem-solving process and quality improvement tools.[15] The Quality Circle movement, which incidentally is still seeing success in Britain's National Health Services, had gotten so much right; what went wrong?

Quality Circles were a bottom-up approach to process improvement. They were legitimized from the top of the organization through the provision of resources in the form of training, facilitators, meeting space and time, policies permitting them access to in-company assistance and executive support. In effect, Quality Circles were told: "Go, run with it!"

Managements that supported Quality Circles in their organizations were by definition liberal and empowering. But something was missing. Quality Circles were about methods improvement rather than sustainable quality. Their formation implied no recognition by management that quality was a problem or needed to be a priority. Thus Quality Circles were born as happy orphans — no parent could be found. There are some clear lessons, two in particular.

Quality improvement needs to be a cause, concern or — to use Joiner's word — an obsession for the *whole* company. It cannot be allowed to become the cause of one individual or the goal of one team. This end will be expressed by the regular gathering and dissemination of data that bear upon quality from both the professional and the customer perspective. Senior management will be as seized by these data as with the financial statements. Second, senior management will retain the responsibility for quality improvement, because management owns the processes by which work is done. At the same time, it will delegate its active pursuit of quality improvement to those most competent to identify opportunities, diagnose effects and remedy performance, namely, front-line practitioners.

There seems to be general agreement between the proponents of Deming's methods [16] and Dr. Juran's [17] as to how these principles play out in practice. I will describe this consensus in my own terms.

The basic quality improvement unit consists of three components which together make up what I call the Quality Improvement Triad:

- A quality improvement or project team

- A superior group or Quality Council

- A facilitator or mentor provided by the superior to assist the project team

The role of Quality Council or superior is played most commonly by senior management, the CEO, Vice Presidents, and Chiefs of Staff. The project team will be a small group of employees — supervisors and practitioners — chosen by the Quality Council from the departments and functions that share in the process targetted for improvement. (See Exhibit 10.7.)

Exhibit 10.7
The Quality Improvement Triad

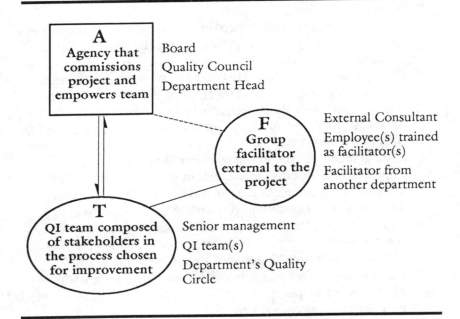

This basic structure needs to be repeated at different levels in the organization. At the senior level, roles A, F and T will be board, a faciliator or mentor from *outside* the hospital, and senior management. When the target process occurs almost exclusively within one department, the project team (T) is called by Juran a QC Circle, and the department head must act as the project team's sponsor (A) and find its facilitator (F) and other resources. Wherever it occurs in the organization, a project team's role is to improve performance and the satisfaction of the customers. Quality Councils and their equivalents have two roles: to support and improve the QI process in the echelons reporting them, and to improve the quality of the service(s) they themselves provide. The latter role tests the value they add to the organization.

Scholtes [18] arranges his hierarchy differently:

QI Council —> Guidance Team —> Project Team

Others would take the role(s) of the Guidance Team into the relevant QI Council. This strategy will become plainer when we outline the roles of the three players we have named.

The QI or Project Team

This is a group of from five to nine members drawn from either a single department (if the process is wholly owned by that department) or the various trades whose work contributes to the cross-departmental process. The composition of the team is more than a matter of egalitarianism or industrial democracy. Recently I was part of a highly educated and — we thought — experienced group of hospital professionals (one physician, two administrators, two QA co-ordinators, two consultants) who were given the task of lessening the waiting time of patients scheduled for admission in an ordinary community hospital. After a series of exercises in problem solving over a three-hour period, the overwhelming problem that was observable at every turn was our lack of competence in the basic tasks we had been assigned: ward clerk, cleaner, transportation orderly, RN, admitting clerk.

There are three roles that are assigned within the project team: leader, recorder and time keeper. The leader is usually a department head chosen by the Quality Council or other authority endorsing the value of the project and authorizing the team to undertake it. The recorder (or team secretary) and the time keeper (whose activity makes members time conscious) are chosen by the team from among its members.

The Quality Council

The Quality Council is in one way similar to a QA committee, in that its central responsibility is for the quality and effectiveness of the QA or (in this case) CQI program. But the Quality Council is far more: it usually has authority over all those whose participation in and co-operation with the project and its solution are likely to be required. Where its rule does not extend, it will usually be able to negotiate the services that the team requires. In some programs, with some projects, a member of the Quality Council may choose or be detailed by the CEO to sit as a member on the project team, to enhance its work and demonstrate the commitment of senior management. Probably every CEO should participate in a CQI project every second year, particularly one with major physician involvement.

The Quality Council should:

- Select the project from among many recommended

- Choose the leader

- Endorse the membership

- Designate the facilitator

- Provide the resources: time, space, library, data gathering, technical assistance

- Provide a written mandate

- Receive regular or stage reports

- Act on its recommendations

- Champion, recognize and, at the project's completion, discharge the team.

The Facilitator or Mentor

The facilitator acts as midwife to the quality improvement project undertaken by the team. She (or he) has three major roles, and these define the sort of person a facilitator needs to be. She must be able to teach. One of her first responsibilities is to provide on-the-job or just-in-time training in quality improvement to the newly formed team. Second, facilitators need to be experts in the group process. While the team is outwardly focussing on the project, subconsciously it is being ravaged by "Group Dynamics 101": form, storm, conform, and perform. Third, the facilitator needs to have the basic technical skills of CQI, in particular, problem solving, data gathering, and knowledge of the Seven Tools (see Chapter 11).

Of all companies, hospitals should have the least difficulty in finding good facilitators within their employee ranks. Teaching, problem solving and non-directive counselling are essential skills in the training and practice of a whole host of professionals. While large companies employ full-time facilitators, community hospitals may prefer to train at one time six to twelve people, selected in conjunction with the hospital's outside CQI mentor, to act in the capacity intermittently.

Facilitators perform their roles directly with the team leader before and after the team's meetings, which they attend as observers and non-participants. Facilitators prepare the leaders for their team meetings; they assist in setting goals and anticipating group needs. Following each meeting — during which they take notes on the process — they debrief the leaders to increase their insights and look at the resources the team is going to need — before the next meeting and beyond.

Facilitators should confer periodically with each other, with the outside mentor (who probably participated in their training), and with the Quality Council. The facilitators become the collective memory and experience of the company-wide program. They share with the mentor responsibility for the development, improvement and regeneration of the program. The mentor "makes it happen" with senior management. The facilitators reward management's commitment with the output of productive quality improvement teams.

10.10
Addendum:
Deming's
Fourteen Points

One of the legendary formulations of the quality improvement movement is Deming's Fourteen Points. They are like Luther's Ninety-five Theses, nailed to the door of the castle church at Wittenberg in 1517, which began the Protestant Reformation. Deming's Points are a challenge, a manifesto, a charter. They call for repentance and a turning from bad practice and exploitive and short-sighted management. This prophetic view is enhanced by the fact that Deming couples his Fourteen Points with the Seven Deadly Diseases:

1. Lack of constancy of purpose

2. Emphasis on short-term profits

3. Evaluation of performance, merit rating or annual review

4. Mobility of top management

5. Running a company of visible figures alone

6. Excessive medical costs

7. Excessive costs of warranty, fuelled by lawyers who work on contingency fees.[19]

Deming added some Thirteen Obstacles [20] which he saw as not quite so serious as the Deadly Diseases. His Fourteen Points are essentially a statement of his philosophy of management. They originate from his early days of work in Japan and have grown in number and changed in their actual wording over the years. The version given in Exhibit 10.8 is from December 1988.[21] The purpose in reproducing them here is more than historical. The Fourteen Points are widely used in introducing CQI to a management team. Executives are encouraged to review them, explore what they might mean in their particular setting, and discuss whether they could or should be adopted in the company or hospital. Walton quotes Deming as saying to the U.S. Agency for International Development: "Export anything to a friendly country, except American management." [22] The Fourteen Points make clear Deming's view that the most urgent need for quality improvement is in the executive offices.

Exhibit 10.8
Deming's Fourteen Points

---

1. Create constancy of purpose toward improvement of product and service, with the aim to become competitive and to stay in business, and to provide jobs.

2. Adopt the new philosophy. We are in a new economic age. Western management must awaken to the challenge, must learn their responsibilities, and take on leadership for change.

3. Cease dependence on inspection to achieve quality. Eliminate the need for inspection on a mass basis by building quality into the product in the first place.

4. End the practice of awarding business on the basis of price tag. Instead, minimize total cost.

5. Improve constantly and forever the system of production and service, to improve quality and productivity, and thus constantly decrease costs.

6. Institute training on the job.

7. Institute leadership. The aim of leadership should be to help people and machines and gadgets to do a better job. Leadership of management is in need of overhaul, as well as leadership of production workers.

8. Drive out fear, so that everyone may work effectively for the company.

9. Break down barriers between departments. People in research, design, sales and production must work as a team, to foresee problems of production and in use that may be encountered with the product or service.

10. Eliminate slogans, exhortations and targets for the work force asking for zero defects and new levels of productivity. Such exhortations only create adversarial relationships, as the bulk of the causes of low quality and low productivity belong to the system and thus lie beyond the power of the work force.

11. (a) Eliminate work standards (quotas) on the factory floor. Substitute leadership.

    (b) Eliminate Management By Objective. Eliminate management by numbers, numerical goals. Substitute leadership.

12. (a) Remove barriers that rob the hourly worker of his right to pride of workmanship. The responsibility of supervisors must be changed from sheer numbers to quality.

    (b) Remove barriers that rob people in management and in engineering of their right to pride of workmanship. This means, *inter alia,* abolishment of the annual or merit rating and of Management By Objective.

13. Institute a vigorous program of education and self-improvement.

14. Put everybody in the company to work to accomplish the transformation. The transformation is everybody's job.

— Scholtes, P. (1988). *The Team Handbook: How to Use Teams to Improve Quality.* Madison, WI: Joiner Associates, p. 2.4.

References

1. GOAL/QPC (1988). *The Memory Jogger: A Pocket Guide of Tools for Continuous Improvement.* Methuen, MA: GOAL/QPC.
2. Walton, M. (1986). *The Deming Management Method.* New York: Putnam.
3. *Ibid.,* p. 13.
4. Ishikawa, K. (1985). *What Is Total Quality Control? The Japanese Way.* Englewood Cliffs, NJ: Prentice-Hall, p. 107.
5. *Ibid.,* p. 19.
6. Massey, M. (1976). What you are is where you were when. (Video). Boulder, CO: Morris Massey Associates.
7. Davis, N.M., Cohen, M.R. *et al.* (1981). *Medication Errors: Cause and Prevention.* Philadelphia: George F. Stickley, p. 17.
8. Barker, K.N. (1969). The effects of an experimental medication system on medication errors and costs. *Am. J. Hosp. Pharm.* 26:325.
9. Ishikawa, *op. cit.* (see Note 4), p. 139.
10. Imai, M. (1986). *Kaizen: The Key to Japan's Competitive Success.* New York: McGraw-Hill, p. 15.
11. *Ibid.*
12. Testimonial, Kanichiro Ishibashi, Chairman and CEO of Bridgestone Co. Ltd.
13. Ishikawa, *op. cit.* (see Note 4), p. 198.
14. Thompson, P. (1982). *Quality Circles: How to Make Them Work in America.* New York: American Management Association.
15. *Ibid.,* p. 105.
16. The Hospital Corporation of America; Joiner Associates; many major corporations, including the 1990 Deming Award winner, Florida Power & Light.
17. The Juran Institute; National Demonstration Project; Harvard Community Health Plan.
18. Scholtes, P. (1988). *The Team Handbook: How to Use Teams to Improve Quality.* Madison, WI: Joiner Associates, pp. 3.7-3.8.
19. Walton, *op. cit.* (see Note 2), p. 89.
20. *Ibid.,* p. 93.
21. Scholtes, *op. cit.,* p. 2.4.
22. Walton, *loc. cit.*

11

The Process and Tools of CQI

11.1
The Improvement Process

In this chapter we move from the broad canvas to a single figure standing in the foreground, from a description of facility-wide total quality management to the step-by-step passage through an improvement project. The second half of the chapter will deal with the process, data and statistical tools employed in continuous quality improvement (CQI). When I began my investigation of quality improvement I believed, naively, that CQI was all about a set of statistical methods that possessed a special, new magic. Of course, this supposition was ridiculous; tools are just tools. What is powerful is the *process* by which an individual or team brings about change.

Readers in CQI will find that each author favours a particular set of defined steps. Berwick *et al.* have twelve [1];

the Hospital Corporation of America has nine [2]; Scholtes has five — or is it twenty-five [3] ? When all the methods are placed side by side, they share a certain logic: (1) projects are initiated; (2) teams spend time investigating the current situation, and propose remedies; (3) they test them, and following satisfactory evaluation, introduce new improvements one at a time. After each implementation, (4) teams reiterate, i.e., return with a new improvement to step 3, *or* they close the project. We will look at each of these phases in turn: initiating, investigating, changing, and reiterating *or* closing.

Team Preparation

Quality improvement projects begin with the selection of an operating problem. It is assumed that problems will be recognized by front-line workers, or be perceived by departments as a result of customer complaints or response to survey. Some writers [4] encourage the search for problems — but perhaps the most important activity in the beginning is that of assuring staff and management that problems can be exposed without fear of reprisal, that nominations are encouraged, and that they will receive response. Line problems will go to department management, and managers will forward to the Quality Council (or senior management) operating problems that are too large or too complex to be addressed within the department. Problems must be nominated with sufficient information to allow the Quality Council to choose among them and to authorize the formation of a project team. CQI authors [5] concur that, when ranking problems for a first project, teams consider as a key criterion the likelihood of success.

Quality Councils are responsible for six activities in this start-up phase:

- Receiving nominations for process improvement or problem solving;

- Deciding on the disposition of these nominations, including the order in which they will be attempted;

- Authorizing the establishment of a quality improvement (QI) team;

- Choosing a team leader and suggesting the team's composition;

- Nominating a facilitator;

- Defining the roles of the Council, facilitator and team, including a written charge, mandate, or terms of reference for the project.

The next key role is that of the facilitator, who essentially guides the team through the process. The facilitator will be responsible for training the team, for briefing and debriefing the leader at each step through the process, and for finding and providing the resources the team needs. Scholtes advises that the initial training or orientation of the group could include:

- Deming's Fourteen Points/Joiner Triangle [*quality - all one team - scientific approach*]

- The scientific approach

- What is a process?

- Customers and vendors

- The 85/15 rule

- How this project fits into our organization's larger effort

- Our partnership with the management team.[6]

Much of this material occurs in the historical account of CQI given in Chapter 10, which could be adapted for team training. However, Scholtes' last two topics, which ground the team's efforts within the context of the company's goals, deserve particular inclusion.

The team leader's tasks are to begin forming the team

through "get-acquainted" exercises, to effect the choice of the other two functionaries (recorder and time keeper), and to lead the team in a discussion of mutual expectations or rules, such as the necessity for regular meeting times, prompt attendance, and courtesy. The obviousness of such rules should not diminish their importance. The following list is attributed to QualTec, the management consulting arm of Florida Power & Light:

- Respect each person
- Question and participate
- Share responsibility
- Attend all meetings on time
- Criticize only ideas, not people
- Listen constructively
- Keep an open mind.[7]

The other necessity in making a start is getting the mandate straight. Whatever the initial form of the charge, mandate, or terms of reference, the team must convert it into a simple *problem statement* (e.g., "Patients scheduled for admission complain about waiting too long in the waiting room before being escorted to their rooms") and later into a *mission statement* (e.g., "Within three months, to reduce by 50% the number of X-ray reports being filed late, according to the *Standards*"). If teams have difficulty in arriving at a simple problem or mission statement, they can take the matter back to whomever gave the mandate, so that the situation is clear to both parties. With a problem statement and a mission statement in hand, the team is ready to begin what Juran calls its diagnostic journey.

Problem Investigation

Quality improvement prescribes a disciplined and logical process for both diagnosing and remedying problems. The sequence of steps is intended to answer the questions: What does the team know or believe now? What are the current facts of the situation and what do they mean? and, How can the process best be improved?

Present Knowledge

The team starts with a problem — or better, the symptoms of a problem — often stated in terms of customer dissatisfaction. It then works backwards to the probable causes. It can use some or all of three strategies: *brainstorming,* in which all team members give their opinions as to what is happening and why; the construction of a *flow chart* to describe, in order, the steps taken in implementing the process behind the problem; and the development of a *cause-and-effect* or "fishbone" diagram, which lists by category causes of malfunction. (Each of these will be described later in this chapter.) These exercises will increase the shared knowledge of the team. In particular, they will demonstrate what the team does not know or cannot agree about, and hence will identify what it needs to know in order to choose an appropriate remedy. For example, teams often discover quite different beliefs among themselves as to how a process is meant to work, and the places in the process where short cuts or errors are frequently made.

Just the Facts

A key aspect of diagnosis is testing or gathering data. Again, this task is approached in a disciplined way. Having determined what the team must know about the process in order to address it, the team must identify which aspects of performance it can measure, then develop the methods and tools to do so and gather the data accordingly. Then it will analyze its data to establish the validity of the causes it proposed. Data can be gathered by survey, by inspection, or by collecting incidents, elapsed times, rejects or returns. Supporters of CQI often commend quality improvement as "management by facts", and several QI tools are used to enable the facts to speak for themselves: *histograms* or bar charts, *run charts* showing scores over time, and *scatter plots* that register the concurrence of two variables.

Choosing a Remedy

CQI teaches people to attack not symptoms but root causes. The Japanese instruct QI teams to ask "why" five times before being satisfied. Thus, the team's tasks at this stage are to identify *root causes* and to develop a *range of strategies* or solutions before choosing the one that will be implemented first. Pareto charts (which separate the "vital few" facts from the many), cause-and-effect diagrams and decision matrices are commonly used to help teams rank and choose remedial strategies.

Process Improvement

In making changes, the password is PDCA (or the Shewhart/ Deming cycle). The team must *plan* — design or map the changes implied by the remedial strategy. Then it implements the changes (*do*) and measures or *checks* the results before *acting* to introduce the revised process. Often remediation is much more complicated than the simple *plan-do-check-act* sequence would suggest. The remedy may need to be tried and reviewed before being introduced under operating conditions. Nor can the team afford to neglect the human side of the equation — resistance to change. QI teams must be sensitive to the fact that, while people may be willing to change, no one likes to *be* changed. Accordingly, teams must enlist the process operators as the agents and owners of change, and make them part of the process of improvement.

The team needs to establish controls or a system of monitoring indicators to show how well the revised process is working, before finally handing the process over to line staff.

Return or Rest

The remedy has now been introduced and has been shown to work — the job is done, right? Not necessarily. Continuous quality improvement is more than the implementation of single improvements. The Shewhart cycle is intended to rotate until all significant problems have been addressed and all available remedies have been put in place. So the successful implementation of one improvement raises the question: What is the next contributory cause on the list? The reason reiteration makes sense is economy. The improvement team is trained and focussed, the diagnosis has been made, the data gathered — in fact, all the preparatory work has been done. Although the gains to be made in tackling subsequent causes may not be as significant as the gains from the first, they will be inexpensive to achieve if done in the context of the first investigation. In addition, each successive improvement should support those implemented earlier.

The closure of a project should follow the final standardization of the process and its handover to its owning and sharing departments. The QI team needs to submit its report and the documentation of the project; the Quality Council, or other superior, must make sure that the team receives public recognition and the individual members personal commendation for their efforts, which are always made over and above their normal workload.

Exhibit 11.1 outlines the steps in the quality improvement process.

Exhibit 11.1
The Quality Improvement Process

Step 1
Team Preparation
- Select a project
- Choose team and leader
- Appoint facilitator
- Orient team
- Define roles
- State problem
- Formulate team mission

Step 5
Close
- Document project
- Give recognition
- Disband team
- Return to #1

Step 2
Problem Investigation
2.1 Identify customer expectations
- Analyze problem symptoms
- Describe current process
- Theorize causes
2.2 Gather data
- Analysis and interpretation
2.3 Establish causes of variation
- Consider alternative solutions
- Choose one for implementation

Step 4
Return or Rest
- Return to 2.3;
  select next ranked
  improvement
  or
- Return to 2.2;
  gather more data
- PDCA

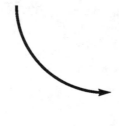

Step 3
Process Improvement
- *Plan:* Improvement
- *Do:* Implement trial test under
  operating conditions
- *Check:* Measure results; evaluate
  effectiveness
- Reiterate "Do" if necessary; address
  resistance to change
- *Act:* Introduce change; establish
  controls to monitor and hold gains

11.2
Quality
Improvement
Tools

Although most of the so-called statistical tools did not originate in Japan, it was the Japanese who put together the most useful ones into a set called the Seven Tools (or Q7) for universal employment in CQI. "Ninety-five per cent of the problems in a company can be solved by the seven tools of QC," writes Ishikawa.[8] Imai also pays tribute to the power of "the seven statistical tools used for. . . analytical problem solving." [9] These tools and others are well and frequently described in North American literature. Of course, it would be too much to expect that all authorities might agree on the same list (or the actual number of the tools!), but the concurrence is fairly close. (See Exhibit 11.2.)

In presenting the CQI tool kit, many variations are possible. Some authors have simply presented their seven,[10] or twelve,[11] or sixteen [12] tools, or have given us the whole collection.[13] Most have tried to relate their preferred tools to the stages or common demands of the improvement process. Scholtes has followed the latter sequence and has introduced his tools in his process narrative. All of these authors have provided illustrations and examples, and for this reason should prove good resources to the reader, as they have to me.

I will here discuss about fifteen tools, according to their purpose or capability, under three major headings:

- Those that *display data* (check sheets, histograms, run charts)

- Those that *analyze or rearrange data* (pie charts, scatter plots, Pareto charts, control charts, stratification)

- Those that record and *portray beliefs or opinions* (flow charts, fishbone diagrams, decision matrices)

Exhibit 11.2
The "Seven Tools" of Quality Improvement

	Ishikawa (1985)	Imai (1986)	Walton (1986)	Berwick et al. (1990)	Leebov & Ersoz (1991)	Total (of 5 Authors)
Pareto chart	x	x	x	x	x	5
Cause-and-effect diagram	x	x	x	x	x	5
Stratification	x			x		2
Check sheet	x	x				2
Histogram	x	x	x	x	x	5
Scatter diagram	x	x	x	x	x	5
Control chart	x	x	x	x	x	5
Graph	and x	x		x		3
Flow chart			x	x	x	3
Run chart†		†	x	†	x	2
Brainstorming				x		1
Data collection				x		1
Total (Recommended Tools)	8	7	7	10	7	

† Run charts are the most frequently named graph.

It is worth adding some means for achieving team participation in theory development and choice: brainstorming, multivoting, the Delphi process, and the nominal group technique.

CQI Tools That Display Data

These are the simplest and therefore the most common of the statistical tools. Their importance is underscored by their inclusion in the Seven Tools recommended by Ishikawa, Imai and Walton.

Check sheets
These are simple tally sheets that record the number of events or quantities as they occur: for example, the number of cars that pass a point during morning rush hour, or the various types of patient (in-patients, day-surgery, clinic out-patients) presenting at the Admitting desk. Check sheets are also used to sort varied data, when they are first recorded in the sequence in which they occur — for example, in a log.

Histograms or bar charts
When people wish to summarize different responses so that their quantities can be compared, they can use a histogram or bar chart. Each response or type of event is represented by a column whose height will be determined by the volume of each. Often the topics of the columns will be unrelated to each other ("Of the 200 respondents, 80 listed as their first choice of recreation watching TV; 45, going to the movies; 35, going to the cottage; and 40, attending sporting events"). At other times the bar topics will be related ("Of the 230 hospitals responding, 12 had boards of more than 30 trustees; 40 had 26-30; 80 had 21-25; 60 had 16-20; 30 had 11-15; and 8 had 10 members or fewer").

An alternative way of portraying related data is the stem-and-leaf plot, which allows a visual arrangement without loss of the original data.[14] (Exhibit 10.2 on page 284 shows data in this form.)

Exhibit 11.3
Histogram

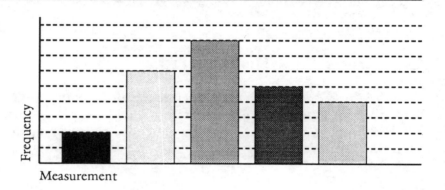

Run charts.
These present volume over time, so that the viewer can notice trends over time and deviations from a mean or norm. In QA, this is the method of choice for reporting performance indicators.

Exhibit 11.4
Run or Trend Chart

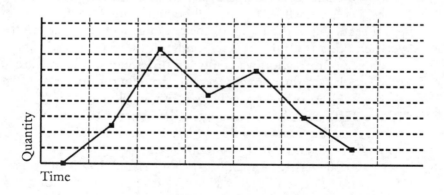

CQI Tools That Analyze Data

Some of the methods or charts for analyzing data are variations on the three methods described above. A Pareto chart is a simple rearrangement of a histogram; a control chart is a modified run chart. A pie chart shows volumes of unrelated data as discrete portions of the whole.

Pie charts
These are much used in the media — for example, to show how national, local or special cause monies are earned and spent. Each slice of the pie represents, by size, the proportion of the whole accounted for by a single source or expenditure. The problem with pie charts is that they are unidimensional. If a team wishes to compare revenue by source with expenditure by beneficiary, then it would need to portray two pies, side by side.

Exhibit 11.5
Pie Chart

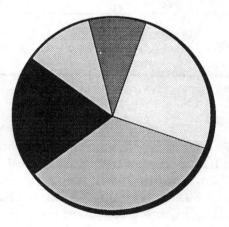

Scatter plots

These are used when a team wishes to correlate data for two factors — for example, individual height with weight, speed with age, length of stay with patient acuity scores. The scatter plot can show either no correlation, positive correlation (i.e., as one variable increases so does the other), or negative correlation (i.e., as one variable increases the other decreases).

Exhibit 11.6
Scatter Plot

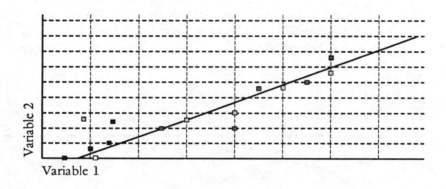

Pareto charts

These were named by Juran, who should be credited with their origin, after the Italian economist Vilfredo Pareto (1848-1923), who discovered that 20% of Italy's population in his day accounted for 80% of its wealth.[15] A Pareto chart is a histogram with two important modifications: the bars will be arranged in descending order from the left, and the diagram will indicate the increasing percentage of the whole, accounted for by the accumulating bars, rising to 100% at the top right of the diagram. A team looking at a histogram can see at a glance which is the major factor in the data, what percentage of the total data it represents, which is the next most important factor, and what percentage of the total factors 1 plus 2 constitute. A Pareto chart helps a team focus on priorities as established by the data.

Exhibit 11.7
Pareto Chart

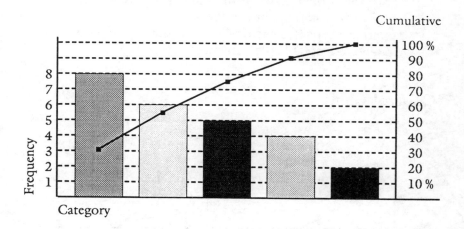

Control charts
These were first developed by Shewhart and are another of the classic Seven Tools. A control chart is a run chart on which are marked an upper and a lower control limit (UCL and LCL). These limits mark the boundaries of the operating process, if it is stable or under control. The sequential readings on the chart should be random about the mean, which is also marked. By looking at the control chart the

team can see (1) whether there are trends (e.g., 7 points moving in one direction or 7 points in succession below or above the mean) and (2) whether there are outliers — readings outside the UCL and LCL. If either (1) or (2) occurs, the team needs to look for special causes. Random variations within the limits are common cause variations and are intrinsic to the process. The UCL and LCL are derived from the process itself, being ±3 standard deviations (SD) from the mean. When the variance is analyzed for a process or effect, 68% of the readings will occur within ±1 SD, 95% within ±2 SD, and 99% ±3 SD. The team should also notice whether performance standards set by the hospital accord with the control chart. If the standards are *inside* the process limits, then staff are in trouble — for they are being asked to operate a process which, when in control, *will* produce or allow unacceptable performance.

Exhibit 11.8
Control Chart

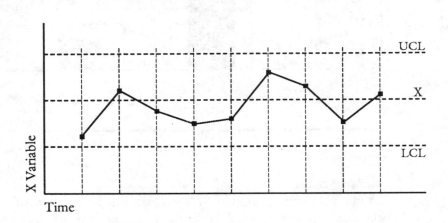

Stratification
This is the separation of data by strata or category.
Sometimes data can hide effects if the categories are too
broad. For example, the average waiting time in Admitting
per day may say little. However, if data were segmented by
time of day throughout the week, they might reveal long
waits between 14:00 and 16:00 and short waits from 17:00
to 21:00. Similarly, average length of stay for the same
complaint might be a meaningless statistic if there are major
contrasts between the treatment modalities — surgical
intervention versus chemotherapy, for example. QI teams
need to be sensitive to their data, and be prepared to collate
or segment them according to the realities they are
measuring.

CQI Tools That Portray Beliefs or Opinions

The first two sets of methods deal with data. This set has to
do with the personal experience and professional insights of
the QI team. It is not a matter of objective versus subjective,
opinion versus reality, because the team's habits and experience are vital to quality improvement.

Flow charts
These are another of the Seven Tools fundamental to quality
improvement. In order to improve a process whose results
have been judged unsatisfactory, it is essential to understand
the process itself. A flow chart is a step-by-step graphic
portrayal of the intended or actual process. It uses common
symbols: *circles* mark start and finish; *diamonds* mark
decision points; *rectangles* indicate a process; and the
document symbol shows form creation and information flow.
    Flow charting is both an essential and an informative
process. Most teams are surprised at the complexity of the
processes they wish to reform. Often they are also surprised
at the difficulty of reaching consensus as to how the process
works, or is meant to work.

Exhibit 11.9
Flow Chart: Handling Correspondence

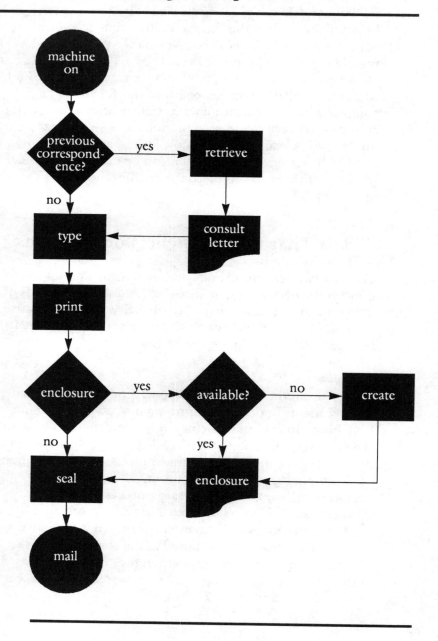

In addition to the common step-by-step or *detailed* flow chart, Scholtes [16] describes and exhibits top-down, workflow and deployment diagrams. *Top-down* flow charts have the merit of setting up the headings of the process horizontally (e.g., Step 1/Plan—> Step 2/Organize) before requiring the actions that are detailed subsequently, below each step title. The major steps thus provide a structure to the chart. *Workflow* charts use a different organizing principle, that of office or facility geography. They follow the path of a document, customer or product from the originating source to the end or outcome of the process. *Deployment* flow charts are keyed off the various agents of the process — e.g., Patient, Admitting Clerk, Emergency Nurse, Secretary, Doctor, Floor Nurse.[17]

Cause-and-effect diagrams

These were devised by Kaoru Ishikawa and are sometimes called by his name or by their shape: "fishbone" diagrams. A cause-and-effect diagram is a graphic representation of the perceived intermediate and root causes of the poor performance scheduled for improvement. Protruding at an angle from the fish's spine are backbones labelled Method, Workforce (Manpower), Material, Measurements and Machinery (the "five Ms"), or Patrons, People, Places, Procedures and Provisions (the "five Ps"). Stated in a box at the fish's head is the particular malfunction, e.g., "Unacceptable Waiting Times in Admitting", "High Incidence of Complete Meal Trays Returned", "High Postsurgical Infection Rate". The construction of a good cause-and-effect diagram is both difficult and time consuming. But if a team is unwilling to spend time hypothesizing probable causes, and searching among them for root causes, appropriate solutions will remain elusive.

Exhibit 11.10
Cause-and-Effect Diagram

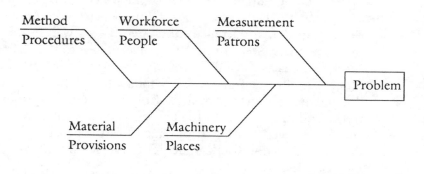

Methods to Ensure Team Participation

Because teams usually comprise people from different strata in the organization, there is always the possibility that the more senior among them will dominate. This is undesirable, and not just for political reasons — the matter is more one of lost competence. Members are nominated to a team because each is perceived to bring to it necessary expertise. If seniority reigns, then much junior but essential competence will be lost to the team. The literature describes several strategies that can help groups to recognize or enhance their functioning as teams: the Delphi process and nominal group technique come from the 1970s; Leebov and Ersoz list focus groups and affinity charts; and Scholtes refers to the Crawford slip method.[18] I am indebted to Paul Plsek for pointing out that all group methods can be summed up in four basic strategies: brainstorming, boarding, multivoting, and the use of decision matrices.

Brainstorming

The oldest, most popular and probably most useful team activity is any method that motivates a group to articulate all its ideas on a given topic. The leader/recorder will encourage the group's creative response by demonstrating an acceptance of all ideas as they are contributed, and discouraging any censorship by group members of ideas as they arise ("That won't work", "We've tried that before", "That's not our job"). Humour and tolerance for the ridiculous will allow the group to use its imagination and propose creative solutions.

Boarding

This method entails the use of storyboards, flipcharts, or "any visual display and organization of ideas that helps people develop a common understanding of a topic." [19] While many authors recommend boarding, Plsek was the first to define it as a basic and generic strategy. In his view, the chief advantages of boarding are that the information is written down for all to see; it focusses team attention, using visual memory to help members follow the discussion. It exposes deep debates and ends trivial ones, and also lets individuals know they have been heard. [20]

Multivoting

This is a discussion and decision process that can enable a team to reach consensus on projects and approaches. It commonly employs an idea-generating exercise such as brainstorming. Ideas may then be ranked and combined (by virtue of affinity) or eliminated (by reason of repetition) before the team takes its first vote. Following the vote, those ideas at the bottom of the list are struck off. The team then moves to a second (or third) vote. The reiteration of ranking and voting promotes consensus on key issues.

Two formal methods of multivoting are the Delphi process and nominal group technique. The latter is specifically designed to preclude domination by seniority (or the loudest voice). It allows everyone to rank-order the group's ideas; then, if polling is not by written ballot, the votes of the "junior" members are taken before those of their seniors.

Matrices

A decision matrix is a useful tool when a team must choose between strategies, or when a Quality Council has to rank proposals for improvement projects. The left side of the matrix will display the alternatives, e.g., an improved pharmacy distribution system, provision of snacks to patients after 17:00, faster turnaround time on lab reports. The columns across the top of the matrix should be labelled with the essential decision criteria, such as "Impact on Customer", "Need for Improvement", "Ease of Implementation", or perhaps "Convenience", "Acceptability", Cost Effectiveness". The deciding agency (a team or Quality Council) will poll its members to arrive at a score (say, from 1 to 3 or 4) for each item. These scores will then be added or multiplied across the criteria to give a cumulative rating, by which indicator the team would then be guided. Although these ratings will be subjective they are team derived, and teams find that objectifying them in this way is helpful. The fewer the criteria, the clearer the reading. The team must also feel that each criterion carries equal weight in relation to the others.

These four methods in no way constitute an exhaustive list. All remind us that, in addition to facts and the scientific approach, CQI requires teamwork and team solutions rather than autocracy and prescription.

References

1. Berwick, D.M., Godfrey, A.B., and Roessner, J. (1990). *Curing Health Care: New Strategies for Quality Improvement.* San Francisco: Jossey-Bass, p. 179.
2. Duncan, R.P., Fleming, E.C., and Gallati, T.G. (1991). Implementing a continuous quality improvement program in a community hospital. *Quality Review Bulletin (QRB) 17*(4 [April]):106-112.
3. Scholtes, P. (1988). *The Team Handbook: How to Use Teams to Improve Quality.* Madison, WI: Joiner Associates, p. 4.30.
4. *Ibid.,* pp. 5.14-5.17; see also Juran, J.M. (1988). *Juran on Leadership for Quality.* New York: Free Press, pp. 47-52.
5. Juran, *ibid.,* p. 52, for example.
6. Scholtes, *op. cit.,* p. 6.
7. QualTec Institute. Palm Beach Gardens, FL.
8. Ishikawa, K. (1985). *What is Total Quality Control? The Japanese Way.* Englewood Cliffs, NJ: Prentice-Hall, p. 197.
9. Imai, M. (1986). *Kaizen: The Key to Japan's Competitive Success.* New York: McGraw Hill, pp. xxiv and 239.
10. Walton, M. (1986). *The Deming Management Method.* New York: Putnam, pp. 96-118.
11. Berwick *et al., op. cit.* (see Note 1), pp. 177-219.
12. Leebov, W. and Ersoz, C.J. (1991). *The Health Care Manager's Guide to Continuous Quality Improvement.* Chicago: American Hospital Association, pp. 99-185.
13. GOAL/QPC (1988). *The Memory Jogger: A Pocket Guide of Tools for Continuous Improvement.* Methuen, MA: GOAL/QPC.
14. Berwick *et al., op. cit.* (see Note 1), p. 207.
15. *Ibid.,* p. 186.
16. Scholtes, *op. cit.* (see Note 3), pp. 2.18-2.19.
17. Leebov & Ersoz, *op. cit.* (see Note 12), p. 148.
18. *Ibid.;* see also Scholtes, *op. cit.,* p. 2.39.
19. Plsek, P.E. (1992). CQI Program, 23 March, pp. 4.3, 4.8. Institute of Health Management, University of Toronto.
20. *Ibid.*

12

The Clinically Augmented CQI Program

12.1
Three Inhibitors

The message of Chapters 10 and 11 is: CQI/TQM is a new species of quality enhancement. It has a distinguished ancestry — a proven track record in manufacturing, information and service fields. It has a special theoretical base and tools and methodologies to produce its effects. In spite of this, hospitals in Canada have circled the dining table: some have sampled the dishes, but few have decided that this is the table that will provide their sustenance today and in the future. In spite of the endorsement of CQI by CCHFA and some provincial ministries of health, there are three reasons for hesitation: cost, hype, and insensitivity. And then there remains the question of CQI's effectiveness.

Cost

Early in February 1992 I was reviewing a compilation of bulletins from the Ontario media. Among them were the following headlines:

> *Health-care changes "a must". Quebec minister warns of a shortfall of at least $2 billion over five years.* (Globe & Mail, *5 February*)
>
> *Mount Sinai lays off 90 employees.* (Global News, *6 February*)
>
> *Joseph Brant Hospital in Burlington announced layoffs of 50 staff to follow from low transfer payments in 1992.* (CHCH NewsRoom Eleven, *6 February*)
>
> *Why health care must be rationed.* (Globe & Mail, *7 February*)
>
> *Health-care administrator resigning.* (Ibid.)
>
> *Five managers and about 10 more people at Network North will get their pink slip before the end of the week.* (CBC Sudbury, *4 February*)
>
> *Crunch at hospitals hits middle managers.* (Toronto Star, *6 February*)
>
> *Some Willett employees endorse wage freeze to help reduce costs.* (Brantford Expositor, *4 February*)
>
> *In Timmins: Dire predictions of hospital closures and service cuts. . . ."* (MCTV, *28 January*)

And, from the United States:

> *U.S. president rejects plan for Canadian-style national health care program, calling it a proven failure.* (CBLT/CBC at Six, *6 February*)

With Canada deep in recession and no end presently in sight, hospitals — the most recession-proof of all companies — are being told to "downsize", to balance their budgets now and accommodate wage and other settlements next year on minuscule increases in income. Hospitals in Ontario are or should be in a survival mode just at the time when CQI/TQM salesmen are offering them a self-actualization program. The discordance between question and answer would appeal to Abraham Maslow.

It is difficult to find reliable figures on the cost of implementing CQI/TQM. In an appendix to his book *Implementing Total Quality Management: An Overview,* Jablonski[1] provides an estimate of the first-year and total three-year costs of introducing CQI/TQM to a company with a 300-person workforce. The educational costs were $562 thousand in the first year and $1.846 million (U.S.) for three years. A multisite university health centre in Michigan has, in 1992, a $1.4 million budget for CQI/TQM implementation, now in its third year. Teaching hospitals in Canada were looking at implementation proposals ranging from $100 thousand to $3 million in 1992. These figures did not include the cost of offsite training including, when necessary, staff replacement costs. For many hospitals, CQI might be the right answer, but it arises at an impossible time.

Hype

Martin Merry commends CQI/TQM to health care executives. He calls it

> *a new paradigm of collaboration and focussed team effort, . . . an organizational transformation, . . . a process [that] must be felt at gut level, . . . a fundamental restructuring of the beliefs and assumptions by which health care provider organizations function. . . .*
>
> *What does it take to accomplish this level of organizational transformation? . . . The answer: nothing less than total commitment from the top of the organization. . . . The board, executive management, and physician leaders must thoughtfully reconsider their institution's vision, values and mission. . . . [It] requires not only a philosophical*

transformation of the mindsets of all employees, it implies a commitment to continuous education for the entire organization.[2]

In what might be a summary statement, Dr. Merry adds:

TQM is not a program that the CEO buys into to improve quality or productivity; it is a way of organizational life that must be lived consistently, day by day.[3]

All of these quotations occur in one four-page article in a respected professional journal. Today, the literature is full of overblown panegyrics whose superlatives and transformational tone bears comparison with year-end automobile sales pitches and furniture store advertisements. The February 1992 issue of the *Quality Review Bulletin* carried an account of the third forum of the National Demonstration Project in Atlanta, Georgia, 31 October – 1 November 1991. The write-up was also replete with the jargon: "organizational commitment", "transformational process", "mission, vision and values", "a way of life and not a program", "not so much a program as an atmosphere", the need for leaders "to walk the talk", transforming "mindsets".[4] At one point, a psychiatrist compared favourably the processes followed in CQI with those used in psychotherapy,[5] and a Blue Cross/Blue Shield vice president summarized his appreciation of CQI as "a way of life, a change of life, a long-term plan, a matter of survival, and a matter of success." [6] But lest the interested buyer imagine that this organizational character transplant comes cheap, its salesmen then insist that chief executives need to mortgage their own time and not look for real results in the organization for three to five years. We should not wonder that many experienced, sober CEOs are staying on the sidelines. They remember the proponents of Management By Objectives, *In Search of Excellence,* and Quality Circles — each proclaiming that their idea was the last word, when in fact is was only the latest word.

Can CQI really be as good as its proponents protest? And will it still be around in 1994?

Insensitivity

Although we probably did many things wrong in starting QA programs from 1984 through 1987, we did get one thing right. From its earliest days, QA organization mirrored that of the host facility, whether a hospital, nursing home, or health unit. CQI comes in demanding organizational change with the assurance: Trust me.

Hospital Peer Review describes the organizational hurdles posed by CQI:

> . . . *Regardless of their opinions about QI's applicability to the health care setting, everyone interviewed by* HPR *agreed that QI is expensive, time-consuming and difficult to implement. Authorities are also concerned that it takes at least five to ten years to achieve the cultural changes needed for QI's success.*[7]

Henry Ford is reputed to have said about his early cars, "Let them have whatever colour they like, so long as it is black." Chief executives who wish to buy CQI/TQM today may feel like the prospective purchasers of Mr. Ford's cars. They can buy a Deming-based model or a Juran Institute model, but the market is provider driven in that the consultant will prescribe what is needed. These inflexible prescriptions are being given at a time when implementation methods for health care are far from perfected. As well, the heavy and expensive emphasis on culture change is reinforced by the consultants' unsubtle reminder that it is senior management's mindset and values that must be changed first.

What is equally galling: nothing the hospital has or operates now in quality is compatible with what CQI/TQM will require. This "so long as it's black" attitude has frustrated proponents of QA in the United States. In an article entitled "Is Traditional Quality Assurance On Its Way Out?", Koska interviewed Homa-Lowry, then president of the National Association of QA Professionals, who voiced the sense of rejection felt by QA professionals across the United States. In their experience, CQI has come in as a new broom.

Its proponents have failed to acknowledge that anyone had done anything about quality before they did. Then to add insult to injury, hospital CEOs who have starved their QA departments have invested thousands of dollars into CQI. [8]

12.2
The Question of Effectiveness

In their haste to supplant QA with CQI/TQM, some proponents have not noticed that the latter also has some weaknesses as a quality strategy for health care. In spite of his exuberance, Merry cautions his readers: "As of this writing, scientific objectivity forces us to reserve final judgement on the ultimate applicability of TQM to health care."[9]

The journal *Hospital Peer Review* agreed: "The jury is still out on how well the quality improvement process. . . will work in American hospitals." [10] The journal interviewed Deborah Green, a quality management consultant who has studied CQI, who was quite blunt in her assessment: "The pure continuous QI approach won't work in health care." [11]

Continuous quality improvement was not designed — and has not been modified — for health care. Why should it then be expected to be sensitive to the needs of this field? As presently taught, CQI (1) underestimates the need for regulation in health care, and (2) is silent concerning clinical activities.

The Need for Regulation

Health care professionals can understand the admonitions in Deming's Fourteen Points: "Cease dependence on inspection" and "Eliminate work standards and numerical quotas", but still they will want and need to maintain quality control practices and double-checks. Imagine a lab without quality control, a department of surgery that is not monitored by a Tissue & Audit committee, or a Radiology department that does not monitor its radiation levels and patient procedures. These QC routines are needed, not by the hospital but as protection for its customers and staff. If they find no place in CQI — and they don't — then they must be integrated into a companion system, which at the moment is called QA.

In a published reply to Berwick's analysis of the QA hospital (A) and the CQI hospital (B), Zusman writes:

> *I believe Dr. Berwick has been too optimistic in describing Hospital B. He has also ignored the value of accumulated years of experience with the traditional system operating in Hospital A. He proposes to substitute an industrial approach to quality that has never been adequately assessed in the medical setting for a time-tested medical approach that has evolved out of many customs (e.g., clinicopathologic conference, autopsy review) and interlocking ethical obligations that health care professions have developed to protect the welfare of their patients.*[12]

CQI's Silence on Clinical Activities

The concept of quality of care is opaque, cloudy, obscure. Customers know only so much. They can talk about pain, disability and disappointment — and of course, their antitheses — yet be uncertain about the connection between their perceptions and sensations and the quality of care they received. Yesterday I had a cavity filled by my dentist. As I write twenty-one hours later, my mouth still feels sensitive. Should I still have this feeling? What kind of job did the dentist do? How long will this filling hold? As the patient, I have no clear idea about the quality of the professional service rendered.

Who would know? Answer: The next dentist who examines me. This introduces the matter of peer review. Not only is the issue of quality obscure to the patient, its assessment by the practitioner is also cloudy. While each professional assesses his or her own work and results as they occur, such assessments are subjective and may be incorrect, insensitive and — a special risk — out of date.

In his afterword to *Curing Health Care*, Garvin refers to both causes of obscurity:

> *The first. . . is the often* murky connection in medical care between *inputs and outputs. In health care, unlike industry, it is not always clear exactly what activities are leading to what clinical results. Cause-and-effect relationships are seldom fully defined, especially when the conditions are rare or are seen infrequently. The second unusual feature of health care is how difficult it may be for the customers [patients] to* distinguish high-quality from low-quality care. *Often health status results are perceived only after a very long time lag; in some cases, differences in technical care quality are simply not discernible by other than highly professional judgement. And even highly professional judgements may differ.*[13]

This silence relative to clinical quality is buttressed by an analysis of the success lists of CQI hospitals, and the projects written up in Berwick's *Curing Health Care*. They share one characteristic — all report improvements in customer processes:

- Waiting times; [14]

- Reductions in grievances, abandoned calls, resource expenditure in total hip replacement; [15]

- Improvement in patient throughput, operating room use, handling of emergency patients.[16]

The *Medical Staff Leader* interviewed Dr. Ersoz, author and Vice President of Medical Affairs in a Pittsburgh hospital.

> *Q: What types of lasting improvements has your hospital been able to achieve through the use of CQI?*

A: Most of our changes have related to turnaround times. I think it is easiest to use CQI to get a handle on improvements in the process of care rendered by laboratories or in medical imaging processes. When you look at the projects that the big hospitals have used CQI for, they haven't been for clinical improvement yet.[17]

12.3
Caveat Emptor

Readers who perceive a change in tone between the high positivism of Chapter 10 and the scepticism with which this chapter began may be wondering whether I have changed my mind between writing the one and beginning the other. Certainly I plead guilty to changing my mind about CQI, but not during the four months in which this book has been written. As I said earlier, I was captured initially by three salient elements of CQI: (1) its understanding of process, (2) its affirmation of the contribution of the workforce, and (3) its offering practical tools to make change possible. But I have had several insights since then that have taken the bloom off the rose.

First, I encountered repeatedly those who needed to buttress their own belief in CQI by converting me to their cause. This still occurs today, and for many adherents of CQI the world is divided into the saved and the unsaved. Those who excite the most anxiety are those who have heard, but have not fully accepted.

Second, I noted — with some irritation, I confess — the habit of CQI advocates commending CQI not because it is good or effective, but because it is *not* QA. QA has all sorts of practical problems but none provides justification for a radically different program.

Third, I became alarmed by the absence of dialogue. The

gods had spoken. CQI/TQM is right; those who question love neither the gods nor quality. I was concerned about CQI's applicability to *all* facilities, about the need to assess a facility's readiness for CQI, about getting the politics right, particularly with the involvement of medical staff and unionized staff. For those who had bought into TQM, these issues were not important. Those who had not, did not wish to discuss them because they knew they were expected to support the cause that had been anointed by CCHFA, CAQHC, the University of Toronto's Health Administration Program and Ontario's Ministry of Health.

Fourth, I became convinced that there is an unintentional lack of rigour and honesty in the reporting of CQI achievements. Laza and Wheaton [18] introduced me to some data comparing Florida Power & Light to other U.S. electric utilities that I would never have suspected from the scores of references to FPL in the CQI/TQM literature and the teaching role it has undertaken for others. Self-reporting by agencies employing CQI is uniformly upbeat, replete with success stories and the universal joy that comes from high participation.

Sixth, and perhaps most damning, I have come to realize that CQI is the solution to no clear and important problem in Canadian health care — neither quality, nor survival. Although it may make us feel better, it provides no definable benefits. In industry, companies can measure their costs of waste, scrap and rework, and their warranty/product return costs. In hospitals, wherever these sorts of measurements are available, they are already in place, and their discrepancies are specifically addressed: e.g., laboratory proficiency, radiation safety, nosocomial infection, environmental safety. If quality is improved in less measurable endeavours, management may not be able to know for sure. Meanwhile, American gurus commend CQI to Canadian health care audiences for survival reasons, by reminding them that the higher quality achieved by CQI will stop patients and their physicians from going uptown to the competing facility. It will, we are assured, enable our CQI hospitals to increase their market share, which in Canada is a blessing guaranteed to strike fear into the chief financial officer's heart.

Where does this odyssey leave the author and the reader? With the Latin motto, "*Caveat emptor* — Let the buyer beware.*"* I will conclude with a caveat from the business world.

In a recent article in the *Harvard Business Review*, Schaffer and Thomson point to the dangers of engaging in quality improvement *activities* instead of focussing QI on *tangible results:*

> *In a 1991 survey of more than 300 electronic companies, sponsored by the American Electronics Association, 73% of the companies reported have a total quality program under way; but of these, 63% had failed to improve quality defects by even as much as 10%. We believe this survey understates the magnitude of the failure of activity-centred programs not only in the quality-conscious electronics industry but across all businesses.[19]*

The authors' prescription is to focus on results:

1. Ask each unit to set and achieve a few ambitious short-term performance goals.

2. Periodically review progress, capture the essential learning, and reformulate strategy.

3. Institutionalize the changes that work — and discard the rest.

4. Create the context and identify the crucial business challenges.[20]

Their opening paragraph describes the alternatives:

> *The performance improvement efforts of many companies have as much impact on operational and financial results as a ceremonial rain dance has on the weather. While some companies constantly improve measurable performance, in many others, managers continue to dance round and round the campfire — exuding faith and dissipating energy.[21]*

12.4
Making Choices

Hospital and medical leaders must make their own choices.
By the time this book is published, I will be assisting a
suburban hospital in Toronto to implement CQI. In spite of
all the negatives I have raised here, I can commend CQI for
five salient reasons:

- Quality assurance as a bottom-up approach has failed to
  engage the commitment of hospital and medical leaders.
  CQI has established an impressive track record of gaining
  executive leadership and sustained commitment.

- While uncertainty continues to be expressed about CQI's
  power to effect change, I am impressed by the balance of
  evidence available. Its insight into what makes things
  work and not work, its system of effecting change and its
  tools, and the promise of political support and adequate
  resources, together may make for a winning hand.

- By their nature, hospitals are towers of Babel that
  function in spite of their divisions of status, language,
  function, skills, and even incentive. CQI's focus on
  processes challenges this isolation and emphasizes the
  role of the team, not that of the specialist.

- CQI's notion of the customer has the potential to
  transform traditional values. The patient really is the one
  who determines quality, and the patient will be served
  only if those who participate in the same processes
  respect the quality needs of their customers, that is,
  those who depend on them.

- If management understands that quality is a function of
  the process which it alone has power to choose, buy,
  support and change, then it is joined inseparably to those

who work the process at the front line. Quality, whether good or poor, is eighty-five per cent of the time a management choice and not an accident of worker skill or motivation. CQI has both understood and explained this equation.

The discussion of which is better, CQI or QA? is sterile. It is like asking a soccer player which foot he wants to play with. His answer is "Both," and if he is a professional, he will have practised intensively with his weaker foot so that he can pass and shoot from either side. So too with quality. An effective quality strategy must combine professional performance with teamwork, bottom-up QA with management-led CQI. But there is one combination that will become popular and should be avoided. I refer to departmental CQI.

In late 1991 the American Hospital Association published Leebov and Ersoz' *Health Care Manager's Guide to Continuous Quality Improvement*. The authors virtually ignore senior management and the quality assurance department and address line managers, for whom the *Guide* is written:

> *Although certain dimensions of your role may vary according to the level of your organization's involvement in quality improvement, you should be implementing quality management practices in your own area and in interactions with your staff and customers. If your institution is not yet involved in an organization-wide quality improvement strategy, do not wait. Educate yourself about quality management and begin to apply what you learn.*[22]

Leebov and Ersoz are democratizing an elite program, taking it out of the hands of the consultants and delivering its tools and strategies to those who manage quality on a daily basis, that is, the department heads.

The Health Care Manager's Guide belongs on the quality-conscious manager's bibliography, but its basic strategy is flawed. CQI is not about making changes with tools and strategies; it is about teams and sharing and interdependence. Unfortunately, many managers excited by CQI will have to go it alone. Their executives may not be able to endorse it, or having done so may opt out, allowing it to go on without their involvement.

But does CQI have to be so expensive and take so long? I believe that the correct answer to both questions is "No." The underlying message of this chapter is that you can get there from here. Facilities can step surely from present QA to future CQI. Some QA practices are compatible with CQI work, indeed some are so essential they will survive CQI. Quality will never be free, but it need not be expensive. Probably CQI practice can be learned on the job, one step at a time, rather than through mass and intensive indoctrination. While CQI will not ultimately succeed if the CEO and medical leaders do not come on board, much work can begin at the departmental and managerial levels, as Leebov and Ersoz suggest.

12.5
Changing
Behaviour

A strong feature of the CQI/TQM literature is the insistence on attitude change within the company. This is referred to as culture change and the development of new value systems and attitudes towards the customer and the employee. The length of time estimated for full implementation and the prescription of training for all levels of management and, sometimes, all employees, is premised on the slowness with which a corporate culture and the company's habits and traditions will change. Thus most of Year 1 is spent in the indoctrination of all levels, in addition to a handful of pilot

QA projects. It seems foolhardy for one author with no supporting literature to oppose this overwhelming consensus, but I do, and do so for empirical reasons.

When I entered the Ph.D. program in adult education at the University of Toronto, I knew that the way to change a person's behaviour was through his or her attitude. By the time I was through, I appreciated the tenuousness of the link between attitude and behaviour and the decisiveness of social or organizational structure. For the last fifteen years all my practice has been based on the recognition that doing things is so much more certain than wanting to do them. The person who does has, even if only for the moment, overcome his or her sense of incompetence, resistance to what is new, and the countervailing forces in the social environment. But what about the person's attitudes and values? They will follow and support the competent practice of the new skill or behaviour. People handle naturally the potential dissonances between practice and values. If they can *do* they will *value;* if they value and cannot do, their new values will soon be extinguished.

In 1987 I advised hospitals to employ the Adult Learning Model (ALM) — a generic strategy for accomplishing organizational change — in introducing quality assurance. The ALM is just as relevant at this juncture. It advises those who would accomplish change to

1. *Start where people are,*

2. *Introduce the new as a modification of the old,*

3. *Introduce the new as a series of single and reasonable demands that build to the total behaviour desired,*

4. *Involve a Steering Committee, which represents both*
   - *top-level support, and*
   - *the level of management expected to get the job done. . . .*[23]

Because the ALM has the word "learning" in its name, some people have failed to notice that it is an action strategy.

It calls on the agent of change to help participants do better what they do now and then take a series of action steps, each preceded by some just-in-time training. I believe this is the practical, sensible and effective way for hospitals to assimilate CQI/TQM.

12.6
Practical Steps
from QA to CQI

If proponents of QA and CQI can get away from criticizing and characterizing each other and talking about hype and "bad apples",[24] they may discover some common ground.

In this text we have acknowledged three central weaknesses of our best QA:

- It is strong on measurement but weak on improvement.

- QA's proponents (myself included) have tended to patronize patients and their views.

- QA is department specific: quality is what happens within "my" cell; what happens outside it is not "my" business.

Fortunately, CQI can supply ready correctives for each of these points:

- *CQI is all about improvement.* It investigates why things don't work and finds ways to make them work.

- *In CQI the customer is god.* There is also the realization that everyone has a customer, whether the patient or someone who serves the patient.

- *CQI looks at whole processes,* including customer processes like being admitted, or visiting the out-patient department.

On the other hand, QA has its proven strengths which tend to occur at points where CQI is weak, silent or untested:

- First, QA is in place, not new, threatening or costly;

- Second, it takes seriously the concurrent monitoring (QC) of vulnerable systems of care and service — what CQI calls inspection or checking;

- Third, it has developed expertise in the assessment of the technical/professional aspects of care, where CQI is silent; and

- Fourth, it is a comprehensive system of public accountability.

Our contention is that today's QA can be greatly improved by the employment of ideas and methods from CQI. But we can go farther: holding firmly to QA, we can incorporate CQI's most important and effective strategies.

Described below are the "series of single and reasonable demands" or practical steps that a hospital or its QA committee can introduce to move the management of quality from an accounting to an improvement mode:

A. Get the key players on side.

1. Identify customers, their expectations and satisfaction.

2. Identify and map the major processes owned and shared by the department.

3. "Manage by facts": Learn the Seven Tools.

4. In a departmental project, employ the CQI process and Shewhart cycle.

5. Participate in a *shared* (cross-functional) CQI project.

B. Structure the facility-wide program.

Strategy A
Get the Key Players On Side

I have "lettered" this Strategy A rather than numbering it, because it can occur at any time in the passage from QA to CQI. It does not need to occur before Step 1 but probably should happen before Step 5, when CQI moves out of the orbit of the department to address cross-functional processes.

Similarly, all the key players — board, senior management and medical staff — need not come on side together. The journey to CQI can begin with the first manager who wishes to orient his or her department more directly towards the customer and bring on board the improvement process and CQI tools. However, individual initiatives have a higher likelihood of success where there is a CQI champion in senior management.

Presentations to the board, management and medical officers should occur at retreats or special meetings, rather than at or before business meetings of the board. They could cover most of the material of Chapter 10, with local and national health care information to put CQI in an immediate context. (See Strategy B, below.)

Strategy 1
Identify the Customer

Readers may remember our earlier insistence, in Chapter 4, that no QA program was complete without the department's gathering and reporting patient satisfaction data. This direction is formalized by demanding that departments identify three client/customer dimensions:

- First, who are the department's actual customers? — that is, the people or departments immediately served by its processes or products. The laboratories, for example, would name as their primary customers the physicians who order the tests, and patients only if their staff draw blood or collect other specimens.

- Second, the department needs to articulate their clients' expectations. Staff can begin with what they think they would want if they were customers of the department. But this can only be preliminary to hearing from the customers themselves. The department would need to use open-ended questions in interviews with, or focus groups for, patients or other clients.

- Third, the department can poll its customers on a regular basis to ascertain their level of satisfaction with its performance in meeting their expectations or needs.

Departments will find that they cannot do only Step 1 and then move on. As long as they are involved in or oriented to CQI, they will keep returning to their customers, their expectations and satisfaction.

Strategy 2
Identify Major Processes

TQM gurus like to point out that quality improvement is not a program but a process, and focusses not on outcome but on process. Step 2 says that it is time to get serious about the processes used or the ways in which the department does its work.

Departments can *own* processes, in that sixty-five per cent of their operation is done within or by the department. They can *share* processes if they contribute twenty to forty per cent of the work, or *participate* in them if their contribution is twenty per cent or less. In this second strategy, departments will first identify the processes they own, then those they share. Then they should describe each process by means of a flow chart, beginning with their supplier and ending with the customer.

In Steps 1 and 2, departments are changing the focus of their quality program from principal functions and important components to customer satisfaction and professional practice (processes of care, service, production).

Strategy 3
Learn the Seven Tools

Unlike the other numbered steps, this is a learning and not an action strategy. It is preparatory to the department's first voyage of process improvement. But learning need not occur in rows or depend on outside faculty. Instead, the QI team or QC Circle can assemble popular and accessible texts that have good descriptions of CQI tools — GOAL/QPC,[25] Berwick *et al.*,[26] Leebov and Ersoz,[27] Scholtes,[28] and Walton.[29] The tools can be divided up, one to each member, to master and explain at a future meeting, with department data for demonstration purposes. The tools I have found most useful fall naturally into pairs:

- Brainstorming and cause-and-effect diagrams
- Histograms and Pareto charts
- Run charts and control charts

It is more important for each team member to master one tool than to learn them all. In fact, it is important that teams not feel threatened by tools, statistics or cycles.

Strategy 4
Put Out to Sea

All roads lead to Rome; in CQI, everything leads to appropriate change, to service improvement. The hospital's QA committee should, in this step, encourage departments to undertake their maiden voyage in CQI. Each should take a simple and important process that it owns and move through the improvement steps: team preparation, problem investigation, process improvement, and closure or reiteration. The QA committee will, if possible, provide a process helper to play the facilitator role. At least it will have an observer, so that the team's learning can be applied to other projects.

After the first round of projects, QA committees can introduce process improvement as an *annual* demand of the QA program for all departments.

Strategy 5
Cross-Functional Process Improvement

This last action strategy is an extension of the one that preceded it — completing a departmental QI project. Cross-functional projects may have to wait for success within departments and the deployment of experienced facilitators. Six or more cross-functional projects running concurrently would characterize a well-functioning CQI/TQM program in its first year.

Strategy B
Structure the Facility-Wide Program

Again, this step is lettered and not numbered because there is no right time to do it within the sequence of numbered steps. Presumably it should occur before Step 5. If the facility intends to make a comprehensive and long-term commitment to quality improvement, there are four tasks that need to be accomplished:

- The establishment and orientation of the hospital's Quality Council, with membership and terms of reference.

- The establishment of a process by which cross-functional quality improvement projects can be proposed to the Council for its endorsement and delegated to a team leader of its choosing.

- The recruitment and training of in-house QI facilitators.

- The selection of an external mentor for the facility's CQI program.

Exhibit 12.1 outlines these seven transitional strategies from today's QA to tomorrow's CQI.

Exhibit 12.1
From QA to CQI — Seven Strategies

Strategy A — Get Key Players On Side
- Board
- Management
- Medical staff

Strategy 1 — Identify Customers
Identify:
- External/internal customers
- Their expectations
- Their satisfaction with our service

Strategy 2 — Identify Processes
Identify:
- The major processes owned by the department
- The processes the department shares/participates in

Strategy 3 — Learn the Seven Tools
- Flow charts
- Histograms and Pareto charts
- Cause-and-effect diagrams
- Brainstorming
- Run charts and control charts

Strategy 4 — First (Departmental) Project
Implement the QI process: and the Shewhart cycle:
- Prepare
- Investigate
- Improve
- Close

- Plan
- Do
- Check
- Act

Strategy 5 — Participate in a Shared (Cross-Functional) QI Project

Strategy B — Structure the Facility-Wide Program
- Orient and train the hospital's Quality Council
- Establish process for generating QI projects
- Recruit and train QI facilitators
- Select outside mentor

---

12. 7
In Search of a
Complementary
Model

It is time to pull together the various strands of argument that we have reviewed. Chapters 10 and 11 describe CQI/TQM as a practical and successful program, well grounded in theory, armed with useful strategies, respectful of work and workers, and important because it answers sensibly hitherto unanswered questions.

This chapter began with a review of the reasons why many hospital leaders find CQI an unpalatable choice. In answer to the question: Do you have to buy the whole package? We answered No. CQI is divisible, and its strategies can be used at various levels in an organization. Exhibit 12.1 described seven transitional steps that would allow a facility to adopt the central elements of CQI — customers, processes, tools and teams — one at a time, while the QA vehicle continued along the road.

Sections 2 and 3 of this chapter called on evidence and testimony from many quarters to support the contention that CQI also has its feet of clay. Notwithstanding the Canadian Council (CCHFA), Joint Commission (JCAHO), ministries of health and commissions and panels, CQI may not be a complete or the complete quality program for health care. Instead, Canadian health care has in QA and CQI two flawed quality programs.

The task of this section is to convince the reader that QA and CQI can be put together in such a way as to complement each other — to feature the strengths, and cover the weaknesses, of each.

Building the Model

Certain constructs in both the PIER and CQI models define the function of the department or program. In the PIER model it is mission, principal functions, important components, and indicators. In CQI the functions of a department are established with reference to the customers, customers' expectations, and the processes owned and shared by the department. If we were to take the strongest components from both models, the definition of *function* might look like this:

- Mission

- Customers

- Customers' expectations

- Major processes owned and shared

- Professional standards

The last item requires explanation. Indicators are developed with reference to performance standards. Our thought is to target particularly the professional/technical standards *not* recognizable from the client's perspective.

Evaluation of performance is an important aspect of both quality models. It occurs in the PIER framework through the evaluation of data from patients, audits, indicators, and external agencies. In CQI, evaluation occurs at three levels: first and most essentially, at the level of the ultimate customer, often an external client; second, the internal customers of the department; third, the department itself and its assessment of the effectiveness of the processes it operates. If, once again, the complementary model were to draw on the strengths of both, *evaluation* would probably be undertaken with reference to:

- Satisfaction of needs and expectations of (1) external and (2) internal customers;

- Professional satisfaction as validated by (1) concurrent data on performance indicators, (2) criterion-referenced audits, focussed studies and data-based reviews, and (3) inspection reports from external agencies.

The complementary model stands to benefit from the marriage of the strengths of both models in this area.

The third and final phase addressed by both models is that of response to data or *improvement*. In the PIER formula, the "R" stands for remedy, reaudit and report. In CQI the diagnostic journey is followed by the remedial journey, implementation and holding the gains. As this is the strong suit of CQI, most of its components will find a place in the complementary model, which concludes with the responsibility to report progress and project completion:

- Diagnose

- Improve — PDCA

- Reiterate

- Report

This shopping from two stalls is illustrated in Exhibit 12.2 in which the goods on offer from QA and CQI are shown in the outside columns and those (marked with an asterisk) chosen by the complementary model are shown in the centre.

In the complementary model we have attempted to capture five elements:

1. An openness to the patient as customer;

2. A sense of responsibility to the department's internal customers;

3. Responsibility for monitoring and improving the opaque aspects of performance — the technical and professional components;

4. Effective strategies of improvement;

5. Accountability to those who answer to the community and the taxpayers.

Exhibit 12.2
Quality Management in Health Facilities

PIER Model	Complementary Model	CQI Model
1. Function		
Mission*	Mission	
	Customers	Customers*
	Customers' expectations	Customers' expectations*
Principal functions Important components	Processes owned and shared	Processes owned* and shared*
Performance standards*	Professional standards	
2. Evaluation		
Patients	Customer satisfaction	Customer satisfaction*
Audits: • Criterion* • Focussed studies* • Data-based*	Professional satisfaction via audits	
Indicators*	Performance indicators	
External agencies*	External review	
3. Improvement		
Remedy	Diagnose	Diagnose*
	Improve	Remedy — PDCA*
	Implement	Implement*
Reaudit	Reiterate	Reiterate*
Report*	Report	

*Elements employed in the Complementary Model.

We have seated the model in the line department only because this is the hospital's prevailing structure. Program and matrix organizations are more compatible with quality improvement, and probably will be more used in the future. Meanwhile, CQI will help make department walls more permeable, and cross-functional QI teams increase the joint ownership of processes and hospital goals.

The next section provides a simple statement of the complementary model of quality management for health facilities.

12.8
The Clinically Augmented CQI Program

I have called this complementary model the clinically augmented CQI program or CA/CQI in recognition of the facts that:

- Health care does well to adopt CQI, a program developed in Japan and well tested in North America. It is effective in continually improving products and service and is in tune with our times in relation to the customer and the worker; but

- Health care needs to reaffirm its need to monitor (QC), validate, investigate and improve clinical performance (QA) by means of audit and other traditional and effective means.

- Neither current QA nor the CQI that has so far reached us from the United States completely answers the need for quality management in Canadian health facilities in the mid-1990s. QA is clearly inadequate at three points:

operating entirely within departments, it supports division; it largely ignores patient perception; and it has a poor record of actually improving performance.

- CQI, on the other hand, is weak at the point of technical/ professional performance; is not notable for its concurrent monitoring of major systems; and seems to be accountable only to itself.

Both the QA and the CQI camps need the strengths of the other model to complement their own product. The model could be called an integrated or combined model; I have chosen to call it complementary, and have set it up with five action components: *mission, identification, evaluation, improvement,* and *reporting (MIEIR)*.

Mission
The department's quality management program should begin with a simple mission or role statement, which declares its obligation to provide stipulated services to meet the needs and exceed the expectations of identified customer groups.

Identification
Rather than identify its principal functions and important components, as it would in the PIER model, the department should identify: (1) its external customers, if any, its main internal customers and — if they are not the same as either of the first two — the end users of any processes to which it contributes; (2) the major processes the department owns, shares and participates in; and (3) the essential professional standards the department intends to meet. These will generally relate to patient-centred, high-volume, high-risk or problem-prone activities.

Evaluation

The department will evaluate its performance in three respects: (1) through the monthly monitoring and reporting of its risk and leading indicators, and the annual review of the data behind the numbers; (2) customer satisfaction with the care or service processes it operates; and (3) the auditing/peer review of the professional components of service.

Improvement

Departments will recognize the imperative to improve processes yielding unsatisfactory data and will aim to improve the process rather than work on the outliers. Second, they have a mandate to seize important opportunities to make improvements even though customer satisfaction scores may be acceptable. Process improvement should be used to address both service or delivery processes and clinical or technical practice, and will follow the sequence of CQI/TQM: diagnosis, remedy, implementation, reiteration.

Reporting

Quality improvement may require a different reporting format and frequency (no less than quarterly) than those of QA, but departments must maintain records of their continuing quest for quality and be accountable to senior administration. Quality program reports should be generic enough to carry indicator and audit reports from QA and efforts in and results of improvement projects in which the department played a significant role.

Exhibit 12.3 summarizes these steps.

Exhibit 12.3
The Clinically Augmented CQI Program: A Complementary Model (MIEIR)

Mission

The development by staff of a mission statement declaring
- the department's customers, and
- the projects/programs offered to meet their needs

Identification

- Customers (external/internal)
- Processes (owned/shared)
- Professional performance standards

Evaluation

- Customer satisfaction
- Process effectiveness
- Professional practice (audit/peer review, performance indicators, external review)

Improvement

- Service performance
- Technical practice

Reporting

- Quality accountability
- Implemented change

12.9
Conclusion:
Quality Systems
in Perspective

When the Canadian Council on Hospital Accreditation introduced quality assurance to hospitals in 1983, an important question was: What happens now to quality control? The faddists said that of course it had been superceded by QA. But as people's understanding of QA matured they found within the QA process an honourable and essential place for QC.

Today, now that CQI has arrived, the important question is: What happens to QA/QC? The disciples say: QA is dead; long live CQI. But the counsel of this chapter and probably the field is that QA/QC retains distinct values and should be allowed to thrive within the CQI environment and practice.

By 1996 there will be a new quality system, as yet unnamed. The question then will be: What happens to CQI/QA/QC now that Q4 has appeared? Its adherents will say that CQI/QA/QC represents little but old dry bones. But the more mature will recognize the valid contribution all three still have to offer the field.

As long as quality systems continue to change in health care from time to time, we will know that quality remains high on society's agenda. And apart from love, what else should humanity strive for?

References

1. Jablonski, J.R. (1991). *Implementing Total Quality Management: An Overview*. San Diego: Pfeiffer.
2. Merry, M.D. (1991). Illusion vs. reality: TQM beyond the yellow brick road. *Healthcare Executive* 6(2 [March/April]):18-21. Quoted passages taken from pp. 18-20.
3. *Ibid.*, p. 20.
4. Report (1992). Meeting update: National Demonstration Projects, 3rd Annual National Forum on Quality Improvement in Health Care. *Quality Review Bulletin (QRB)* 18(2 [Feb.]):66-73.
5. *Ibid.*, p. 71.
6. *Ibid.*, p. 70.
7. Special report on QA and quality improvement (1990). *Hospital Peer Review* 15(2 [Feb.]):23-24.
8. Koska, M.T. (1991). Is traditional quality assurance on its way out? *Trustee* 13(Sept.):23.
9. Merry, *op. cit.* (see Note 2), p.21.
10. Special report, *op. cit.* (see Note 7), p. 23.
11. *Ibid.*, p. 25.
12. Zusman, J. (1990). A letter and reply: Peer review and quality management. *QRB* 16(12[Dec.]):418.
13. Garvin, D.A. (1990). "Afterword." In: Berwick, D.M., Godfrey, A.B. and Roessner, J., *Curing Health Care: New Strategies for Quality Improvement*. San Francisco: Jossey-Bass, p. 160.
14. Warner, T. (1991). Implementing continous quality improvement in a hospital. *Business Quarterly 56* (2[Autumn]): 42-45.
15. Schurman, D.P. (1991). Continuous quality improvement: Perspectives and experiences of CEOs of Canadian hospitals. *CJQHC* 9(1 [Nov.]):6.
16. Hassen, P. (1991). Continuous quality improvement: The experience of St. Joseph's Health Centre. *CJQHC* 9(1 [Nov.]):3-4.
17. Interview (1992). Clara Jean Ersoz, MD. *Medical Staff Leader* 21(1[Jan.]):7.
18. Laza, R.W. and Wheaton, P.L. (1990). Recognizing the pitfalls of total quality management. *Public Utilities Fortnightly* (12 April):17-21. (See page 17 especially.)

19. Schaffer, R.H. and Thomson, H.A. (1992). Successful change programs begin with results. *Harvard Business Review* 70(1 [Jan.-Feb.]):80-89. (Passage quoted appears on p. 81.)

20. *Ibid.,* p. 89.

21. *Ibid.,* p. 80.

22. Leebov, W. and Ersoz, C.J. (1991). *The Health Care Manager's Guide to Continuous Quality Improvement.* Chicago: American Hospital Association, p. 15.

23. Wilson, C.R.M. (1987). *Hospital-wide Quality Assurance: Models for Implementation and Development.* Toronto: W.B. Saunders, p. 37.

24. Berwick, D.M. (1989). Continuous improvement as an ideal in health care. *New England Journal of Medicine* 320(1 [5 Jan.]):53-56.

25. GOAL/QPC (1988). *The Memory Jogger: A Pocket Guide to Tools for Continuous Improvement.* Methuen: GOAL/QPC, 13 Branch Street, Methuen, MA 01844.

26. Berwick *et al., op. cit.* (see Note 13).

27. Leebov & Ersoz, *op. cit.* (see Note 22).

28. Scholtes, P.R. (1988). *The Team Handbook.* Madison, WI: Joiner Associates.

29. Walton, M. (1986). *The Deming Management Method.* New York: Putnam.

Index

All acronyms used in this text have been glossed and cross-referenced in the index.

A

C

F

G

H

I

J

K

L

O

P

Q

S

T

Christopher Wilson

Christopher Wilson is an educator who teaches and consults in health care governance and quality assurance in Canada and the United Kingdom.

Prior to establishing his own practice in 1992, Wilson gained extensive experience in hospitals first in the United States and in Canada before joining the staff of the Ontario Hospital Association in 1978. During his 14 years with the OHA, Wilson acted as a management consultant to small hospitals in the province, helping to design workable models for quality and service effectiveness.

Dr. Wilson was educated in Law at Cambridge University, Theology at the Episcopal Theological School in Cambridge, Massachusetts, and Adult Education at the University of Toronto. He received his Ph.D. from the Ontario Institute for Studies in Education in 1977. In 1992 he was appointed an Honorary Fellow of Manchester University for his work in quality assurance.

Wilson is widely published. In addition to more than 50 articles published in scholarly and professional journals, he has written four monographs for different agencies and three books: *Hospital-wide Quality Assurance* (1987), *Governing With Distinction* (1988), and *New On Board* (1991).